LOSING IT!

It's Not What You Eat But What You Don't Eat That Matters!

Julie and Martin Carrick

First Edition published 2019 by

2QT Limited (Publishing)
Settle, North Yorkshire BD24 9RH United Kingdom

Printed by Ingramsparks

Cover image: J & M Carrick

Disclaimer

This book is based on the authors' personal experiences and any suggestions or advice expressed or implied is intended for information only and is NOT given as professional medical/health related advice nor intended to treat, cure or diagnose any medical/health related condition. It in no way constitutes or replaces professional advice or recommendations. If you have a health problem, medical emergency, or a general health question, we always recommend you should consult your doctor.

A CIP catalogue record for this book is available
from the British Library

ISBN - 978-1-913071-39-4

Contents

Before We Started Our New Lifestyle!

February 2018

MARTIN

JULIE

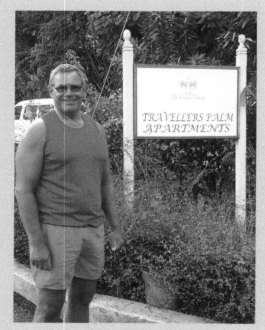

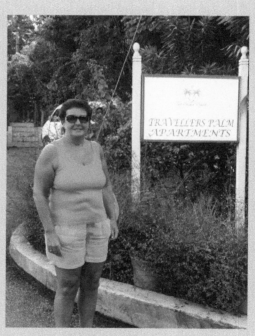

18 stone 7 lbs, 259 lbs, 117 kgs

16 stone 13 lbs, 237 lbs, 107 kgs

Our Success

September / October 2019

MARTIN

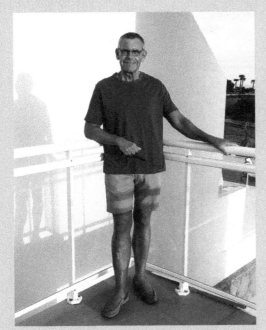

13 stone 7 lbs, 189 lbs, 86 kgs

JULIE

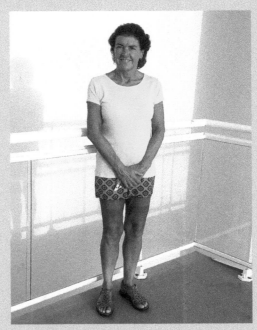

9 stone 13lbs, 139 lbs, 63 kgs

Chapter 1:
Introduction

Allow me to introduce my wife and myself.

We are Julie and Martin Carrick, 60 and 62 years old respectively. Over the last eighteen months we have changed our lives dramatically. I have lost 5 stones in weight, I used to be a XXL shirt size, I am now an M; my waist was 42 inches, it is now 32 inches. Julie has lost 7 stones in weight, she used to be a 20/22-dress size, she is now an 8/10, her waist was 38 inches, size 20. She is now a size 8 in shorts/ trousers.

We are not celebrities or famous in any way. Neither are we nutritionists or experts in the fields of food, dieting, health or fitness.

We are, or were, very frustrated people who had been on diets or health regimes for most of our adult lives. More importantly, we are just everyday normal people who have found a way to change our lives through the food we now eat. The fact that we aren't celebrities attempting to endorse the latest 'fad' diet or 'regime', I hope, makes this book more credible.

We have, however, carried out extensive research into nutrition, diet, health and exercise over the last eighteen months but this book has been written solely based on our own personal experiences, experiments, successes and the failures we have encountered during this time. This doesn't make us experts or make us qualified to make any medical, nutritional or any other claims. The contents of this book are based on our opinions, our personal experience and from the occasional pearls of wisdom we actually found to be true, slipped in along the way.

It is simply a selection of our recipes and how we have utilised the foods we have allowed ourselves to eat in order to become slimmer and healthier people, without a lot of the common pitfalls usually associated with diets and fitness regimes. We have explained what and how we've achieved this, but with very little scientific data. We sincerely hope you enjoy reading about our journey and that you can all experience the same success as we have enjoyed!

Julie was a police officer and was medically retired some years ago following a bad road traffic accident and was subsequently found to have Non-Hodgkin's Lymphoma in her bowel. She is a fully qualified holistic therapist in the disciplines of Reflexology, Indian head massage, Aromatherapy, Remedial and Sports massage and Reiki. She is also a fully qualified instructor and assessor in those disciplines.

I was also a police officer. I joined South Yorkshire police cadets in 1974 and retired in 2006.

Both of us are very keen cooks and bakers, and for most of our lives food has played a prominent part. We have always eaten what we considered healthy, made from scratch meals, whole foods, and all the recommended amounts of fruit and vegetables and the low fat recommendations, in our battle to lose the flab. We had some success from time to time, however, we always went back to our old habits, always regaining all the weight we had lost, plus more. They were all very difficult to sustain or completely unsustainable.

Julie was, in fact, a Weight Watchers leader and ran numerous successful classes. The problem was, their programmes were not sustainable for us, personally, and the weight just piled back on. In our opinion, diet companies actually rely on the fact that their members will return to lose their weight again, time and time again. If everyone lost their weight and kept it off, they would never need to return to the classes. Well I'm sure that if that were the case, they would be out of business quite quickly.

All our adult lives, we have been big fans of keeping fit. Julie is a great swimmer; I am a regular gym attender. It was felt, however, that we were both flogging ourselves to death, but achieving very little, apart from still being fat, albeit quite fit. Despite our weight and builds, we also did a fair bit of running. Again we were just fit, fat people. We had truly tried all sorts of diets, ranging from low carbs, high carbs, high protein, calorie counting and all the rest, but had had virtually no real lasting success.

We had reached a point in our lives where we were at our wits ends. We felt fat and certainly looked fat, but not actually acknowledging the fact that we were so overweight. We had no energy, were not sleeping well and everything was an effort. We desperately wanted advice but we were not finding anything sensible, achievable, or that wasn't contradicting other diet advice offered by the so-called 'experts', even government and medical guidelines.

I had been diagnosed with high blood pressure and was taking all the usual medications to control this, plus statins for high cholesterol. Julie was taking statins as well as thyroxine. We were quite unhappy about our 'lot' at a time when we should have been revelling in life and enjoying ourselves. Our confidence was rock bottom and we both agreed it was time to do something, not just drastic, but something very positive and completely different.

Unfortunately we still had this mindset about

eating 'healthily', but the pounds just kept piling on. We were sometimes eating when we weren't even hungry but just because the clock was saying, 'it's time for tea' we still stuffed it down. I'm sure this is ringing a bell with quite a few people reading this.

We watched all the programmes on television about dieting, fitness and health, usually while eating, but the only advice we gathered from these just left us totally confused and even more down about ourselves and our situation. We were still thrashing ourselves in the gym and swimming pool and losing nothing. If anything we were just getting fatter. I know there will people reading this who will be saying things like, "just cut back", "just watch your calories, it's a case of calories in, calories out". We had heard all this advice before, but believe me, until you are in that position, you really don't know how it feels and how unhelpful, for many of us, that advice is.

There is actually a huge amount of evidence circulating around the diet/health industries that suggest that this is not now the case and that diet is far more complicated than a lot of experts realised or understood themselves! It was and is becoming quite apparent that the answer to weight loss is a complete change in lifestyle and the types of food you eat, and not necessarily the amount.

Chapter 2:
The Beginning

Neither of us had any idea where we were going wrong until one day back in 2018.

We were having some work done in our house. The joiner doing the work turned up to take some additional measurements. He had previously been some six weeks previously, however, when he walked in our house, on this occasion, our jaws dropped in amazement. He had lost a fair bit of weight, looked younger, had sparkling eyes and was clearly healthier. He looked fabulous, completely changed, revitalised!

Obviously he was given the third degree about how he had achieved this astonishing change. He told us about a book that outlined a completely radical lifestyle, food-wise, that immediately had us intrigued.

The book was called *The Plant Paradox* by Doctor Stephen Gundry. Dr Gundry is an eminent cardiologist from America and he devised this programme to make people's lives healthier, actually cure and reverse many common medical conditions and reduce invasive surgery that he considered really unnecessary.

Julie read it first and on completing it, promptly announced that she was going to give it 'go'. She encouraged me to read it as well, however, I was extremely sceptical about it being another 'fad diet'. Eventually I agreed to read it when we returned from the holiday we were about to take. Whilst on holiday, all Julie did was talk about what was in the book and how she was going to give it a try for 6 weeks. She was really excited about what she had read and what she was about to embark on. For the first time in ages, she was really positive about beginning a new chapter in hers and hopefully my life.

It took this holiday to actually take a real good look at ourselves, and others around us. The really sad fact was that we, and everyone around us, almost without exception, were massively overweight. I'm not sure if it was the fact we had decided to do something about ourselves, and our future, but we spent a lot of time looking at other people and I think that's when we made the decision that we couldn't remain how we were. It just seemed that the world around us was becoming fatter and unhealthier at a really alarming rate. Us being two more of them!

Chapter 3:
The Preparation

On our return from holiday, I did read the book, which involved a lot of swearing and shouting out phrases like, "have you read this rubbish". I was more than ready to pack it all in there and then. It looked to me like just another other doctor trying to boost his salary by writing a quick fix book about dieting.

This only lasted for about two chapters and things slowly began to make some sense. What I was reading made it very clear that what we were about to do wasn't a diet but a lifelong change in our lifestyle and hopefully a radical change in ourselves, both mentally and physically.

This is why we don't refer to any of what we have achieved as having been on a diet, but a lifestyle programme.

It was definitely a light bulb moment for both of us.

Briefly, to understand the book and his quite radical ideas about eating and lifestyle completely, you must read it for yourselves. *The Plant Paradox* involves eating lots of fresh vegetables, plants, low to almost nil amounts of animal protein, and where eaten, animals should be grass fed or totally pastured. Grass fed animals are those fed entirely on grass alone and not finished on supplements prior to being slaughtered. Pastured poultry is chicken that is not fed on any additional feed but only eats the grubs from the ground and food it can get from its surroundings. This doesn't mean organic. That is a different thing altogether.

Organically raised animals are actually given additional supplements, mostly prior to being slaughtered.

It also means eliminating many foods that are thought by many 'experts' to be healthy. Some of these foods include things like tomatoes, courgettes, squashes, legumes, potatoes, all vegetables from the nightshade family, most grains, pulses, including rice and pasta.

All vegetables should be 100% organic.

Most dairy is not allowed, apart from cheese and milk from Southern Europe. Products made from A2 casein milk, sheep and goat products are also allowed.

Sugar, in all its different forms, also has to be eliminated. This includes honey and other natural syrups like maple syrup.

The programme is designed to eliminate a protein called lectins, which is found in the foods outlined, mainly in the skins and seeds of the vegetables. Lectins apparently have a bad effect on your gut's good bacteria. There is a far more detailed explanation in The Plant Paradox book of what lectins are and what they do to your gut and body. It's well worth reading and understanding what they are. There are also other sources on the internet that explain what they are, but not many explain why they are not good for your guts in as much detail as Dr Gundry's book. His views are quite contradictory to many other experts' current views.

The programme is predominantly designed to repair your gut and allow the good gut buddies (bacteria) to improve, reduce inflammation in your body and help your body heal itself rather than relying on medications that can be in themselves harmful, due to the side effects they have on your body. It isn't intended as a weight loss programme, but more of a complete change in eating habits to become healthy and increase longevity. So basically it's all about addressing what you eat and don't eat in order to make your gut healthy.

A by-product of doing this can, in many cases, make you lose weight. Ironically, if you're a person under weight it can have the opposite effect and bring your body up to a normal healthy weight.

At this point you will probably be thinking that all this is too good to be true. I certainly did,

however, Julie, cajoled me into carrying on with reading and preparing ourselves for what we were about to embark on.

Something that was beginning to dawn on us both now, was that we could read all the books in the world and watch all the TV programmes available, talk and listen to other people's endorsements about their own weight loss and basically just keep putting off the inevitable, which was, if we didn't get off our fat backsides and do something about it ourselves, nobody else was going to do it for us. Unfortunately we couldn't embrace this fully at the time and couldn't fully accept that we were that fat. Believe me we were. Other people would remark that we were just big and we shouldn't be bothered about our size, but be just proud of who we were and carry on with life with our heads held high. We were neither happy nor proud about our size and desperately wanted to do something about it now. Guess what though. Those people were mostly fat people and are still fat people and will probably remain fat people. It's also my guess that they are really unhappy about it, but just unwilling or can't be bothered to do anything about it themselves!

We also think, that if people are truly honest with themselves, if given a choice, they would also like to be slimmer, healthier people.

The simple choice was ours and it's yours as well. We're glad we made the right choice. I've tried many times to explain and even now as I write, to put into words exactly how we feel now, without getting caught up with emotion or just get lost for words. It's impossible. It's truly an unbelievable feeling. We've said many times that if we could actually bottle that feeling, we could be millionaires overnight! It's truly been that amazing. We now walk past people who we've known for years and they don't recognise us anymore.

We had a further study of the book together and began to formulate a plan for the next six weeks. Six weeks is the time suggested to give your body time to shed its toxins caused by bad eating and for your gut buddies to repair your gut and eliminate the bad gut bugs. During that period we emptied our larder of foods we weren't supposed to eat. Of course we ate most of them. Waste not want not. After all, we are from Yorkshire!

We also printed our own copy of the foods we can eat and the foods we couldn't eat so it was easy for quick reference. This is the 'yes'/'no' list. (Ours will follow later.)

Initially, after reaching our goal weights and being asked by a large number of people what we had been eating, we decided to share some of the recipes that we have designed, tried, tested and which helped us lose our weight in order that we can perhaps help others who were finding themselves in the same position that we had been in.

As we began to catalogue these recipes, it became apparent that we actually needed to explain exactly what we did and how we did it.

I eventually lost 5 stone and Julie lost 7 stone.

Chapter 4:
The Plan

So this is what we did.

This isn't a copy or a simplified version of *The Plant Paradox* book. A lot of the foods we eat and things we did are either slightly or very different to those outlined in *The Plant Paradox*. We did, however, follow the general guidelines in relation to what foods and types of foods we could eat and were pretty compliant with *The Plant Paradox* regime. This was due to several reasons.

In the main, it was the unavailability of some foods, but also the cost. We tried to keep it as simple and easy as possible so that everyone can follow it using their local shops and supermarkets.

For instance, we never ate grass fed or pastured meat or poultry. We have rarely eaten anything organic and until recently steered away from all baking and sugar substitute ingredients, either natural or otherwise.

Julie kept a food diary right from the start and she continues to keep it now. This diary has been essential in order to keep us on the right track and also to look back and see what foods may have caused an adverse weight fluctuation or reaction in our bodies. We strongly advise you to do the same. Keep an accurate diary for yourselves, outlining exactly what food you have eaten for the day and list any reactions, either physically or mentally. Also include

any food cravings you have experienced throughout the day, as some foods can actually induce cravings for, either more of the same foods or for some other foods.

This also includes your level of hunger.

To start the programme, you have a three-day body cleanse. This eliminates some toxins and starts to improve the good bacteria in your guts. Actually, it got us in the right frame of mind to continue our plan and eventual journey. More in-depth details of what we ate during this cleanse are in a later paragraph, however, in hindsight, it is an important part of the programme but not necessarily essential.

During this cleanse, it's quite possible to lose several pounds in weight. This is, however, mostly water. It makes you feel slimmer, though, and was a great boost for us to carry on. Towards the end of the cleanse we quickly realised that we had reached our first major hurdle.

The Plant Paradox is written by an American and as previously stated, a lot of the foods and ingredients mentioned in the book are not available in the UK, other than via the internet. Initially that wasn't too important, but as we read up on what to eat in later weeks, where baking is introduced and very different flours are used to replace traditional white and wholemeal flours, we began to scratch our heads somewhat. Yes they are available on the Internet but they are expensive and we are very much into sourcing our food locally. This is for several reasons: one being to support local small businesses.

It was almost impossible to find grass fed meats and pasture raised poultry, despite living in The Yorkshire Dales, believe it or not. There are some sites in the UK that claim to sell grass fed/pastured products, but the prices were, for us, far too expensive. Closer investigation into grass fed animals, did in fact, reveal they do still receive supplementary foods to 'finish' them prior to being slaughtered. For us it was just too much hassle and too expensive.

We found the same problem with organic produce: very expensive and to be completely honest, in most cases, no better than the everyday products sold in the supermarkets. Unfortunately we don't have the room to grow much of our own. We do grow our own rhubarb, strawberries and also a selection of fresh herbs.

During the first three-day cleanse and for subsequent breakfasts, you are supposed to have a green smoothie. Firstly, we didn't own a blender, and secondly, Julie hates smoothies. Something about the texture I think. Broccoli soup works just as well. It's just a hot smoothie! (See recipes and plan later for what we initially ate for our breakfasts.)

Next comes the question regarding what to drink, both alcoholic and otherwise. We haven't drunk alcohol now for nearly twelve years, so that wasn't even a consideration we had to bother about. We have drunk decaf coffee for some time now and tea, black with no sugar, so that was also an advantage for us. You can drink caffeinated coffee, it's just that we drank so much of it; we thought it was maybe a good idea to go decaf. Our sleeping has improved as a consequence.

For those who do drink alcohol, they will need to cut that out completely for the first two weeks. After that you can drink red wine in very small amounts. That is a small glass per night. You can also have a small measure of spirits but that isn't as well. It's one or the other! Beers and lagers aren't allowed.

As for other drinks, all 'soda' type drinks like Coke, including diet and zero versions, are off the menu. This also includes concentrated squashes, even the ones containing no added sugar. Basically these beverages are just full of rubbish that will kill off your good gut buddies (bacteria) and many of the so called 'no added sugar' versions do, in fact, contain hidden sugars and/or artificial sweeteners.

So it's just water, bottled, carbonated, still or just straight from the tap; black tea and coffee, fruit or herbal teas. I can see a lot of you now pulling a face and thinking you can't do that, but you will surprised how quickly you get used to it and how nice some of the fruit and herbal teas are. For us nowadays, the thought of having milk in tea or coffee is just horrible. It just tastes too greasy now. We've recently tried some almond milk in coffee and as far as we are concerned, it just spoils a good cup of coffee. Just save your money and have it black.

By now, I realise that some of you will be thinking that everything I've said up to now is all far too restrictive and time consuming. I promise you that once you're into it, maybe three or four days, you'll actually begin to enjoy it and all that's involved is a little pre-planning regarding shopping and just changing your usual shopping list so that it includes all the foods you will now be eating.

The first six weeks is split into two weeks followed by four weeks. If after six weeks you've reached your goal weight, you can then start to introduce some of the foods you initially had to eliminate. However, a word of warning here.

When you start introducing some of these foods, there's a good chance you will have quite a bad reaction to them. This is because your gut has had a real good chance to begin to heal itself and then when you go back to eating these foods, your gut rebels and tells you it doesn't want it anymore and wants to go back to eating the other foods.

An example of this for us occurred about halfway through our regime. By this time we had been on it for about 5 months. We went away to Greece and began to eat Greek salads that contain a fair bit of cucumber and tomatoes. Twenty minutes or so after eating, we both felt dreadful. We felt very sick, tired and lethargic and were suffering from terrible stomach and headaches. We both initially put this down to either a bug or something we had eaten. The effects lasted about 4 hours, after which they abated somewhat.

After experimenting with different foods over the next few days, we were able to establish that we couldn't now eat fresh tomatoes or cucumbers without having the same reaction to them. We have had further episodes of these reactions, always with the same foods. We later found that we had the same reaction to beans and pulses so we don't eat those anymore either. Funnily enough, tinned tomatoes, especially when cooked in a curry in a pressure cooker, do not have the same effect. Apparently this is down to the fact that the lectins in tomatoes are greatly lessened when cooked in a pressure cooker.

The Plant Paradox book did suggest that this can occur, the sceptic in me initially refusing to believe it. I do now though. These reactions can differ greatly from person to person. Luckily for us, we seem to react similarly to the same foods so it makes things easy for us.

I'm actually only glossing over the details contained in *The Plant Paradox*. The book explains in much greater detail why your gut influences how the rest of your body reacts and works when you consume different foods and when you actually get your gut working properly.

We are not qualified in any way to make any health or weight loss promises or cures. Dr Gundry is and he has used his medical knowledge, research and experience to write the books he has written and make the claims he has made. Again, I suggest that anyone who is really intent on changing their life to read it. It's a very interesting read.

Whilst undergoing our current lifestyle changes and subsequent weight loss we have both carried out a fair amount of research into diet, nutrition and their link with our guts, mind and bodies. This has been via many different sources, including our own doctor, the Internet and numerous books. Believe me, it's a very in depth and complex subject and one that's still in its infancy at

the moment. The experts are still very much divided, some just claiming it all to be a total fad, others seeming to see it as a revolutionary breakthrough into medicine and health for the future. This also includes mental health as well as physical health.

It's because of this uncertainty amongst the 'experts' that we have decided not to go into any great detail about 'microbiomes' and what is actually in your guts and the complex way in how they work and how they regulate so many different sequences and chemical changes within our bodies.

Everything we've written in this book is information derived from the trials and errors we have experienced and practiced and it's just basically a book about the recipes we have made up in order to make the food we eat now more interesting and varied. It also continues to help us keep control of our weight and health.

We still understand how tempting it can be to eat that piece of cake, dessert or favourite bar of chocolate, but having experienced the pitfalls of actually doing that, we now know it's far easier in the long run to just not eat that sort of food any more, remain disciplined and stick to what we know makes us feel good and keeps us the way we are now.

We were amazed at how conflicting the so-called experts' opinions were, however there were several factors that stood out for us and these were factors that seemed to be supported and agreed by most of the experts concerned. These were:

1. Eliminate or cut down on all processed foods and prepare your own from scratch.

2. Eliminate or cut out sugars completely.

3. Cut down vastly on animal protein and consume more plant-based proteins such as nuts, legumes and pulses.

4. Cut down on carbs like white bread, pasta and rice.

5. Eat foods that address the welfare of your gut, which will in turn look after the rest of you.

Well we did all this but also went a step beyond their recommendations. We completely stopped buying pre-prepared meals/foods of any kind and we just made everything from scratch. For some time, before we started our current eating habits, we didn't eat takeaways and only recently started eating out in places where we know we can get the food we now eat and love.

We don't have any sugar at all now, except for a small amount of organic stevia, which we now use in some baking recipes and using ground almonds and coconut flour in place of traditional flour.

Stevia seems to be the most natural, no calorie, no carb sweetener on the market nowadays. It does have a slight aftertaste, but you don't need a lot because by the time you get to try it, your taste buds will have altered so much, that a very small amount tastes so sweet. You can also use it for cooking.

We're still not totally convinced with how natural Stevia is. It does undergo a process to abstract the sweetness from it and there appears to be more and more evidence evolving that, even though it's supposed to be calorie and carbohydrate free, your brain actually thinks it's sugar and causes your body to start the same response it has when you eat ordinary sugar! (More about this and our experience with stevia towards the end of the book.)

Our animal protein consumption is now very small and we eat a lot of nuts, nut butters and hemp seeds for our protein sources. We also try and eat more fish, such as sardines and mackerel because of the good oil content. Fresh salmon is also a source, of which we eat a lot.

We've vastly cut down on carbohydrates (carbs) and we get our only source of carbs from leafy greens and some salad foods. A full list of our choices will follow later. So-called experts still try and tell us that carbohydrates are essential for our bodies. That isn't actually the case and there is plenty of evidence out there to suggest otherwise. We do eat some carbs, but get them from veggies.

Because of the diary that Julie was completing on a daily basis, we were able to establish which foods suited our guts and which had an adverse reaction, which we could then eliminate and move on to something else.

As I've previously stated, this book is not a copy of The Plant Paradox book, but a story of how we've adapted that programme to work for us and subsequently write a number of easy recipes that have worked for us and we think will work for you as well. That also means in terms of affordability and availability as well as simplicity.

We've tried to stay within the parameters of the compliant and non-compliant foods outlined in The Plant Paradox and we just eat food from our own list of compliant foods.

These recipes have been tried and tested by us, and some of our family and friends. They are amazed at the amount of food we eat and how tasty it is. We have often been accused of serving up food that we have cooked especially for our guests. That isn't true though and they've simply been eating the food we now eat. That's one of the reasons that each recipe is accompanied by a photograph to show how much there is to eat. So, yes, there are some restrictions on some foods, but virtually none with the foods you are allowed to eat.

One exception here is animal protein. This is restricted to 100 grams at each meal, although it is possible to miss that at lunchtime and then have 200 grams later that day, say for supper.

Another is cheese. Cheese is restricted to just 25 grams at any one serving, but only once in a day.

An additional word here about cheese. If possible, eat goats or sheep cheese. It's far more easily digested and most people are far more tolerant of it. Cheese is a strange food really because some people are far more tolerant to it than others. Some seem to pile on the weight whilst eating it. Others don't. It's very easy to eat too much. It's something you will have to work out for yourselves. (Remember to keep your diary.)

I realise, by this time, some of you will be thinking, 'how many calories are we allowed to have per day?' Well the good news is, there isn't any calorie counting. The only weighing to be done is with your protein consumption.

A mention here about oils and fats. Oils such as vegetable, rapeseed, corn and any other oils processed from grains are not allowed.

Oils that are permitted are: extra virgin olive oil, refined olive oil for cooking, avocado oil, coconut oil, sesame oil, hemp seed oil and many of the oils derived from nuts. A more in depth list will follow. There is a suggestion that extra virgin olive oil, EVOO, is actually a healer and we consume great amounts on our salads. We also consume the other recommended oils in quite large quantities. It took some time to get it in our heads that consuming these oils is in fact good for you. We also have small amounts of butter, either salted or unsalted. This is not on a regular basis as it is a dairy product. We actually use EVOO or coconut oil more often now in baking. Refined olive oil is fine for cooking so long as you don't let it burn. After all the Mediterraneans have been using it for centuries with no problems.

Around 5 months into the programme, we suddenly realised how much weight we had lost and how very much different we felt mentally and physically. We had lost around 4 stone each by this time. Our wardrobes contained clothes that no longer fitted and we had to embark on a clothes-shopping spree to replace them all. Strangely enough, this included shoes! We had actually lost weight off our feet.

We seemed to have masses of energy and were doing things that previously, had been uncomfortable, difficult and tiring. Riding our motorcycle was one of them. Another one was travelling by plane. It was so much easier and comfortable now. Just carrying out jobs around the home and garden were effortless and we could work all day and not feel absolutely worn out like we had done before.

Our training was going exceptionally well and despite the weight loss, we had virtually lost none of our previous strength or muscle tone. In fact, we were a bit stronger in both the gym and swimming pool.

We continued to eat the same way and by November 2018, I had reached 13 and a half stone and Julie had reached 10 stone. We're still that weight today and intend to stay that way. Julie is now the weight she was when I first met her nearly forty years ago and I honestly can't remember weighing 13 and a half stone. I must have been that weight at some stage in my teens, early teens, because I'm sure when I was roughly 16/17 I was already up to about 16 stone.

It's difficult to imagine, now, eating any differently and going back to eating rubbish and the so-called 'healthy' foods we used to eat. It's really exciting coming up with new ideas and recipes with the foods that are 'compliant', or foods that we, at least, deem to be compliant and safe and healthy for us.

So here we go with our list of foods we now eat and a list of foods we completely avoid at all costs.

The 'yes' foods are all foods we find suit us and our bodies, and this is now our 'store cupboard' list. There are some foods on the 'no' list we haven't tried at all and some we have re-introduced in order to check their effect on us. Again use your diary to keep a check on what works for you.

Give it a good read before deciding it's 'too difficult and confusing'. Look around your cupboards and larders. You may be surprised to find that you have already got a few of the 'yes' foods already.

If you have quite a lot of the 'no' foods, don't throw them away. Either eat them until you have fully decided to embark on your new eating plan, or if you have made that decision already, give them to your family or if you're feeling charitable, a food bank.

The lists are quite extensive so there's plenty to choose from.

Chapter 5:
Your store cupboard changes!

STORE CUPBOARD - YES - FOOD

By the way, apart from the protein sources, i.e. meat, nuts and dairy which should be weighed, and resistant starches, which are to be eaten in moderation, everything else is unlimited. So gorge away on your veggies and reap their benefits!

Oils	Olive oil. Both extra virgin for salad dressings, drizzling over cooked meats and veggies, and refined olive oil for cooking. Coconut oil. Avocado oil. All nut oils for salad dressings, drizzling over cooked meats and veggies. Sesame oil. We use it for a dressing on stir fries. We use a lot of oil, especially olive oil. Don't use it sparingly.
Sweeteners	Stevia. Erythritol. Xylitol. Remember what I've already said about sweeteners!
Nuts and seeds	Macadamia nuts, almonds, pecan nuts, walnuts, pistachios, pine nuts, coconut and unsweetened coconut milk and cream, chestnuts, hazelnuts, flaxseed, sesame seeds, Brazil nuts and hemp seeds (preferably hulled). Apparently hemp seeds are one of the few plant-based protein sources containing all the essential amino acids your body needs.

NOTE:	Peanuts and cashew nuts are not allowed. Peanuts are a legume and don't grow on trees and can have severe reactions in people. Cashew nuts are also not truly nuts, even though they grow on a tree. They actually grow under a flower/bud on a tree and don't have the same sort of kernel as true nuts.
Olives	All olives except those stuffed with peppers or chillies.
Dark chocolate	Needs to be 75% cocoa solids and above. 25 grams per day. (Our favourite is Aldi 85%. It's really smooth and doesn't leave you wanting more. It's also pre-wrapped in individual 25-gram bars!)
Vinegar	All vinegars including balsamic, but read the labels to make sure there is no added sugars in any of them.
Herbs and seasonings	All herbs and seasonings, including curry powders. Check pre-mixed curry powders as some contain rice flour. We buy East End spices, which we find very good.
Flours	Coconut flour, almond flour, cassava flour is also ok, but we found it isn't the easiest flour to bake with and does have a strange taste. It's also quite high in carbs so we've left it alone. Ground almonds and almond flour have been our mainstay. Ground almonds are a lot finer than almond flour.
Ice cream	There are some commercial brands of ice cream around that boast of being sugar and dairy free, but in the main we found that they do contain sugar. There are some recipes later on in this book outlining what we have created. They do, however, contain some stevia. Worth trying later on in your programme.

Dairy products	25 grams of cheese per day, preferably goats or sheep's cheese. Blue cheese is a better choice as the blue veining is good for your gut bacteria. Feta cheese. We use Aldi as it's good quality and made from sheep and goats milk. Butter. Yogurt. Goat or sheep's is best. Also there's a brand called CoYo which is made from coconut milk. It's quite expensive but very tasty. Double cream. Full fat crème fraîche. Sour cream. Mascarpone cheese. Cream cheese. Natural unsweetened kefir. Check the labels for added ingredients and sugars.
Wines and spirits	Champagne and red wine, one 6 oz glass per day, or, 1oz of spirit. (Only after the first two weeks, but preferably stay free of alcohol until after six weeks.)
Fish	100 grams twice a day of any fresh fish or canned fish. Canned has to be in olive oil, brine or water. No tomatoes or other oils or sauces. Canned tuna, salmon, sardines and mackerel are great because, generally, they come in just the right portion sizes for one person, give or take a gram, which certainly makes preparing easy! All shellfish, again, not pre-prepared in any sauces.

Fruit	Avocado. Try and eat at least half of one everyday.
	All berries that are in season e.g. strawberries, raspberries, blueberries and blackberries.
	We grow our own rhubarb and have eaten that in season with a small amount of stevia and it's been fine with us and not as sour as we remembered. A good sign that our sweet tooth has diminished greatly.
	Fresh lemons are also good for adding to tuna salads as a seasoning.
Vegetables	Cruciferous vegetables. These include broccoli, brussels sprouts, cauliflower, all cabbage, kale, bok choy, Swiss chard.
	Chinese leaves.
	Spinach - We use fresh in salads and the frozen type that's frozen in small balls. With the small portions, it's really easy to use, because you can get out just the right amount you need, either put it in curries or casseroles, or defrost it in the microwave, squeeze out any excess water and use it to have with eggs in one form or another for breakfast.
	Garlic.
	Fresh ginger.
	Onions, red and white, spring onions or shallots.
	All types of salad leaves.
	Watercress.
	Radishes, including Asian radish.
	Fennel.
	Carrots.
	Mushrooms.
	Raw beetroot, grated on salads. We do use pickled beetroot but check it doesn't have any sugar in the pickling liquor.
	Chicory.

Vegetables continued	Okra, also known as ladies fingers.
	All fresh herbs.
	Celery.
	Swedes (makes great chips).
	Tinned tomatoes, only after six weeks.
	(You may find you cannot tolerate tomatoes by this time. A sign that you are intolerant to tomatoes is that you feel very bloated, a little bit sick and either suffer from constipation or diarrhoea. Or you have slight flu symptoms e.g. hot or cold sweats.
	This goes for other foods as well. If you have any of these symptoms omit the foods you think it might be. Check your diary!)
Resistant Starches	In moderation only - maybe once or twice a week.
	Sweet potatoes.
	Parsnips.
	Celeriac (makes great chips).
Poultry	100 grams twice a day
	Chicken.
	Turkey / Duck / Goose.
	All game birds.
	Eggs (no more than 2 a day).
Meat	100 grams twice a day.
	Beef.
	Lamb.
	Pork.

Meat continued	All game.
	No shop bought sausages, bacon or burgers unless you're absolutely sure what's in them. They shouldn't contain cereal or fillers of any kind. It's best to make your own. We have included a recipe later for pork burgers.
	Just a note about meat. We don't skin our chicken, except in curries. We eat it. We also don't over trim our meat of its fat. Fat is flavour. This isn't a low fat diet.
Plant based Protein	Some Quorn products. Check the labels because some contain sugar and a lot of preservatives.
	Hemp seed tofu, if you can find it. There are recipes on the Internet on how to make it yourself.
	Some veggie burgers. (Again check the labels for cereal and sugars.)
	We aren't vegetarians so aren't very clued up with plant based protein sources. Soybean tofu isn't allowed though, because of the process involved in making it. It's not a particularly natural product as far as we can see. Vegetarians can eat lentils and beans and we imagine you could replace the weights for meats with lentils and beans etc.
	It's suggested that all beans and lentils etc. should be canned or at least cooked in a pressure cooker in order to remove as many lectins as possible. Sorry but you'll just have to make your own judgement here as we've just not eaten that much in the way of legumes over the last eighteen months. However we have experimented with a selection of beans and pulses. Each time we have tried them we have both suffered from bloating, flatulence, sickness and sometimes hot or cold sweats. Whether vegetarian or not, if you suffer from any of these symptoms, you need to check your daily diary to pinpoint the source and then eliminate them if necessary for 7 days. If you try them again and get the same reaction, you need to avoid them completely. Individually, by experimenting with different foods, you will find out what does and does not suit you, thereby creating your own tailor made diet.

THE - NO - FOOD LIST

These are all foods that need to be avoided or eliminated from your diet completely. Some might appear to be quite controversial. They are, however, foods that contain a lot of lectins, or are highly processed or have high carbs or high sugar content.

Refined starchy foods	Pasta, wholemeal, brown and white.
	Rice of any kind, brown or white.
	Potatoes and potato products like crisps.
	All dairy milk. (Unsweetened almond and coconut milk is allowed after the first two weeks.)
	All bread and bread products, including naan and other Asian type breads.
	Pastry and products using pastry.
	Any flours made from grains. This includes spelt and corn flour.
	Quinoa, couscous, bulgur wheat and pearl barley.
	Biscuits, crackers (except our flaxseed crackers).
	Ryvita etc.
	Breakfast cereals.
	This includes porridge oats, muesli, granola, breakfast bars, biscuits and other so called 'healthy' foods.
	All sugars, including sweeteners (Some Stevia is allowed, but you will have to judge for yourselves if it agrees with you.)
	All diet drinks, sodas and drinks claiming to have 'no added sugar.'

Vegetables	Tomatoes, cucumbers, peas, sugar snap peas and mangetout, green beans, broad beans, chickpeas, soy and soy products like tofu and textured vegetable protein products.
	All beans and lentils.
	(Vegetarians will need to use lentils and beans for their protein sources and experiment with which works best for them. You may find that you are actually intolerant to some of them, especially if they leave you bloated, windy and slightly 'off' after eating them.)
	Aubergine.
	Peppers of any colour.
	Courgettes, all squashes like butternut squash and fresh chillies.
Nuts and seeds	Pumpkin seeds, sunflower seeds, chia, peanuts and cashew nuts.
Fruit	All fruit except in season berries. (Sparingly for the first six weeks. In our case, it was until we achieved our goal weight. We now still use them sparingly.)
	This includes:
	melons, bananas, oranges, peaches, nectarines, grapefruit, pears and apples. This avoidance of fruit is, at least, for the first six weeks. After that you can experiment by slowly adding some fruit, but only a bit at a time. Fruit is essentially sugar in a different form. Some people find that when they start adding too much back in their diets, the weight starts going back on.
Dairy products	All milk.
	All yogurts, including so-called low fat and ones including grains and fruits, except full fat, natural Greek Yogurt.

Keep to the 25 grams of cheese. If you feel you can't stick to that small amount, you are probably best avoiding it completely, at least until you've lost your weight or feel more in control.

Cottage cheese.

Any sort of protein powders used either for supplementation or meal replacements.

Oils

Rapeseed oil.

Peanut oil (groundnut).

Corn, sunflower or supermarket 'vegetable ' oil (usually rapeseed).

Margarine and all other so-called 'healthy spreads'.

Meat

All processed meat products.

These are items like: sausage, chorizo, salami and all shop bought pre-cooked meats, such as, boiled ham, corned beef etc. All the sort of items you would probably buy for your normal packed lunches really. Instead use your own cold cuts left over from roasts from the night before. One of our favourites is lightly toasted mixed nuts, left to cool and then mixed in with your salad.

Either avoid bacon completely, or, restrict it as much as possible. We do use some lardons in our cabbage carbonara recipe, but only a small amount. Bacon contains a lot of nitrates and preservatives, which are not good for your bodies.

I recently went on a butchering course and part of this course was for us to make our own bacon using a dry cured 'natural' method.

The ingredients were:

A piece of belly pork that was placed in an airtight container or plastic bag. A mixture of salt, then saltpetre was added to the belly pork which we were allowed to take home, to place in the fridge for a week, turning, mixing the pork and curing mix, daily. By the end of the week, the pork had taken on that pink colour that bacon tends to have and there was quite a lot of strange looking liquid in the bottom of the bag. The meat is then washed and then hung to dry for a few days. That's your bacon!

The interesting fact here, though, is saltpetre has to be bought via a special permit because of its use in explosives etc. The ratio of salt and saltpetre has to be measured very carefully because saltpetre is actually dangerous to consume!

Most supermarket bought bacon, apparently, contains much more adverse ingredients than just the two I have outlined. Anyway, your choice. Certainly food for thought though. A mushroom omelette for breakfast begins to sound very much more attractive, I think!

In Summary

As you will see, there isn't a lot of fruit in there, or starchy carbs. Nor the cereals we are told are 'healthy' for us. They are essentially all sugars, or at least they are after they have been through your digestive system, sugar which your body will want to use as energy.

When it's used up, your body will then crave more carb type foods, to go through the same process and thus ignoring your stored fat. Any excess calories from carbs are then converting into fat and stored by your body. Again, your body will then crave the carbs to begin the same process. It's a bit of a catch-22 situation, unfortunately.

The general idea is, that you get your body to start burning your fat and the fat/oil you eat for its fuel, not carbohydrates.

During our research I read an article that compared carbohydrates and fats used as fuel in our bodies. Sugar, a carbohydrate was placed in a bowl. Oil was placed in a separate bowl and both were set alight. The sugar lit up instantly and burnt off almost immediately and went out. It would only keep alight by adding more sugar, more calories. The oil/ fat burnt very slowly and wouldn't need topping up for a much longer time. It was therefore being used/ burnt more efficiently.

All a bit technical, but I hope you get the message. Cut out the sugars and carbs and your body will adapt and burn your fat. When your body is burning fat it doesn't seem to create the same cravings as it does when burning carbs. In fact you will start to crave food like salads and green vegetables etc.

There is also very little dairy. That's because dairy contains lactose, which is also a form of sugar. A large proportion of the world does, in fact, have difficulty in digesting dairy because of having lactose intolerance. You may be surprised to find that you are one of those.

Enough of the science now, let's get going.

First - **a word of caution**. We would strongly suggest that if you are suffering from any serious illnesses or currently receiving treatment from hospitals or a doctor, then you should speak to them about what your intentions are.

We didn't, we continued with the medications we were taking. We just decided to start the programme and then spoke to the doctor at a later date.

It's important to stress here that we had been monitoring our own blood pressures at the doctors surgery and found they had vastly reduced. As a result of this we made appointments to see the doctor and we were taken off the medication we were taking.

The doctor was actually very interested and impressed with our success at that stage. She questioned us as to what we were doing and her response was to just keep up with the good work.

We were subsequently given further appointments for the following months, where we were given blood tests to monitor our progress. Everything improved, and we were taken off other medication we had both been taking for high cholesterol.

Chapter 6:
Make a shopping list

Make sure you've been shopping and bought all your compliant veggies, nuts and oils, canned fish and stocked up your freezer with frozen fish (not battered or breadcrumbed), chicken and meat. Frozen broccoli and cauliflower are also great freezer ingredients for quick meals. I think you can even buy frozen cabbage these days. If it helps you, buy it. I've mentioned previously about frozen spinach balls - a great ingredient for portion control. Just make sure if you're defrosting before use, defrost it in a sieve over the sink to drain any liquid from it. Otherwise just chuck it in curries or our recipes for broths and stews, straight from frozen. We generally use about two to three balls per person.

Make sure you have some avocados for your salads. Buy some soft for eating immediately and some that are hard and which will ripen over the next few days. Eat at least half a day or even a whole one.

If you're working, be prepared to pack up your meals the night before plus any snacks of vegetables or nuts you may feel you need.

Make sure that by now, all the temptations in your cupboards, fridge and freezers, have been removed. This means removing all ready meals, pies, pizzas, etc. that you will not be eating.

I realise that if you have families/children living with you, it's going to be slightly more difficult to achieve this, but just talk to them beforehand and explain exactly what you're about to embark upon. Let them know how

serious you are about becoming slim and healthy and how your current weight and health is affecting you. Also invite them to join you in your journey, especially if they are in a similar situation.

Don't make your shopping trips a chore.

Make a list of food you need and try and stick to your list. Don't be tempted to buy anything you shouldn't be eating.

Again explain to your partners and family that you are going to stick with this for six weeks and you would really like their support and that support will start with what food you are going to be buying over the next month and a half. You never know, they might even join you. Even better!

If you are keen to eat organically, well by all

means, go down that line. That includes meat and fish as well as vegetables. We didn't, for a number or reasons I won't go into at this stage, but just shopped at our local Booths and Aldi supermarkets for fruit, vegetables, meat and fish. We just chose what looked the best on the day and also what was the cheapest. You will get through a lot of veggies and salad ingredients so make things easy, both for you and your wallets! We bought all our nuts, seeds, stevia, and flours such as almond and coconut flour from Grape Tree. They have an excellent choice and have some very reasonable offers. They also sell dried herbs, spices, some vitamins and minerals supplements. You can also shop on line with Grape Tree and have your orders delivered to your door. We cannot speak too highly of them.

There will be occasions when you will need to pack some food up, especially if you are working or travelling. Over the last year and a half we've tried all sorts of containers and re-sealable bags etc. and finally found that Lakeland sell the best for both quality and price, in our opinion. You can shop on line with them also and, at the time of publication, it's free delivery for orders over £50.00, I believe.

They are very helpful and informative about loads of food related goods and accessories like blenders and food processors. We eventually bought our blender there and wouldn't be without it now. The other good thing about Lakeland is that if you're not happy with your purchase, you can return it, no questions or quibbles!

A quick mention here about coffee. We drank and still drink a vast amount of coffee. That was one of the reasons we went decaf some years ago. We found a decent instant coffee we both liked and have stuck with that brand for a good while now.

Since starting our new healthy lifestyle journey, we have been drinking our coffee black. During this time we have looked for a good coffee that tastes good black. A good few of the ones on the market, both instant and from pod or coffee machines, have that bitter after taste. We came across Nespresso pod machines and really liked their coffees. They tend to be very smooth and flavoursome and the decaf versions are produced using a 'Swiss' method, which I think means the caffeine is removed using a water washing method, rather than using chemicals.

We quickly moved on from one of their original machines and onto their latest 'Vertuo' machine. This has slightly bigger pods and produces a bigger cup of coffee. It makes excellent black coffee and has a really creamy 'crema' (froth).

They are a great company to deal with and their 'boutique' stores are well worth a visit if you're interested or like your coffee. They let you try all their range and the staff are really 'up' on their knowledge of the different coffees they sell. You can order on line with them and most of the time they deliver next day.

Although we have mentioned a number of retailers in this book, none of them have been involved in the writing of this book or have influenced us in anyway in what we have written. These are our choices and opinions only.

We have included a number of photographs from various stores showing the produce and products they sell. Some of the photographs show the prices of these products. These photographs are for illustration purposes only and the prices are subject to change without notice.

Chapter 7:
The three-day cleanse

Here's how we started with the three-day cleanse. What follows is taken from the diary that Julie has kept throughout. Don't be fazed by this 'cleanse' period. It's not difficult and you will feel better by the end of three days. Stick with it. Keep your diary!

THREE-DAY CLEANSE.

Day 1		
	Breakfast	20 grams mixed nuts.
	Snack	20 grams mixed nuts.
	Lunch.	Mixed salad of celery, lettuce, radishes, mushrooms, olives, half an avocado and dressed with olive oil.
	Dinner	Sautéed broccoli, carrots, onions, mushrooms and celery. 100 grams of roast chicken thigh meat.
		1 square of 85% dark chocolate. (We had this mistakenly, but still recorded it in our diary).
Day 2		
	Breakfast	20 grams mixed nuts.
	Lunch	Mixed salad of lettuce, celery, mushrooms, radish and carrots. Half an avocado and 6 olives. 60 grams of tuna, plus 15 grams of leftover roast chicken. Dressed with 1 tablespoon of olive oil.
	Dinner	Fennel, cabbage, onions, garlic and ginger, sautéed in coconut oil with 100 grams of pan-fried cod.
	Snack	20 grams mixed nuts.
Day 3		
	Breakfast	20 grams mixed nuts.
		Half an avocado.

Day 3 cont/..	Lunch	Broccoli soup, plus 50 grams of pan-fried salmon.
	Dinner	Sautéed broccoli, cauliflower, onions, ginger and garlic, plus 170 grams of roast chicken leg. (The larger amount of chicken, was to make up the protein levels to around 200 grams each for this day).

As you will see, the three day cleanse is quite restrictive. During this period you will feel hungry and you may also feel a little weak and maybe have some mild flu-like symptoms. Sorry, but this is just your body adjusting to its new foods and eliminating any toxins that have built up over the years.

We found it was easy to keep busy during these first three days so that we weren't thinking about food or hunger. Looking back, however, we really didn't think the three days were that bad at all. We actually didn't have any side effects at all and after the third day felt full of energy and ready to start the next two weeks. We actually continued training during our cleanse and really didn't suffer at all.

If you do have any reactions/side affects, just try to take it a little easy until they pass. They will pass, I promise you and you will start to feel amazing.

Drink plenty of water, black tea and coffee, along with fruit and herbal teas. Not only will this help to fill you, but will keep you hydrated as well. Funnily enough, fizzy water does seem to make you feel full as well. It's probably the gas in it. Anything that helps along the way is good with us!

After the cleanse, weigh yourself and record it in your diary. I'm sure you will have lost a few pounds if you have stuck with it. It's mainly water at this stage, but you should already be feeling a great deal better.

Chapter 8:
The next two weeks

The next stage is the first two weeks of your six-week eating plan. This isn't as restrictive as the cleanse, but there's no alcohol allowed yet.

Keep weighing your protein and remember you can eat as much leafy greens and salad ingredients as you want. Have a snack on 30-50 grams of raw nuts but don't over do them. It's just a small handful.

You will see by now that we have nuts and yogurt for our breakfasts plus a further snack of nuts later on in the day. Well that snack can be in the form of nut butter, spread on lettuce, cabbage leaves or celery. Again don't overdo the nut butters. It's maybe just two teaspoons only. The nuts or nut butter will keep you full, though, until your next meal.

Weigh yourself weekly and record your weight and any other observations i.e. hunger levels, any cravings and generally how you feel, in your diary.

What follows is just an example of one day's eating during the first two weeks copied from Julie's diary.

Example of a one-day menu

Breakfast	20 grams mixed nuts.
	50 grams sheep's yoghurt.
Lunch	20 grams mixed nuts.
	Half an avocado, lettuce, radishes, celery and olives, dressed with 1 tablespoon of olive oil.
Dinner	Sautéed broccoli, cauliflower, onions, ginger and garlic. 100 grams of roast chicken.

Please don't think you need to stick to our example. It's just there to help you know what we were eating and to give you ideas as to what you can do yourself. Experiment with the foods on the 'yes' list. Apart from your protein choices, everything else is unlimited.

If you're good with smoothies, go for them for breakfast. Our recipe is one that we've sort of borrowed and adapted to suit our tastes. Invent your own, from foods on the 'yes' list. We don't have them now. Just not our cup of tea really.

It's also worth bearing in mind here, a quick note about smoothies. Whilst doing our research, we discovered that there is evidence that shows that smoothies are not that good for you or your guts, which is quite contradictory to a lot of other 'experts' advice. The reason is, that you actually miss out some parts of the digestive process. The first being chewing or mastication in the mouth. This actually triggers off responses in your gut, which basically says, 'get ready, there's some grub coming'. It sort of acts as a warning system. The smoothie then enters the stomach but doesn't stay there long as it's already been broken down into a liquid in the blender. It then quickly enters the small intestine, where it doesn't stay long enough for all the goodness to be extracted and absorbed into your body. This is, again, because it's all in liquid form, which, in turn, can cause diarrhoea in some people!

I'm sure there is far more science involved here than we are qualified to make a proper opinion on. Have a go yourselves and you decide.

Chapter 9:
Just four more weeks!

So far, so good?

This is the start of your next four weeks. Continue to weigh yourselves weekly and record this and make any observations in your diaries.

You can introduce alcohol now if you really want/need to. I would suggest, however, if you just don't want to drink at this stage, well don't. Remember though, you can't save up your daily glass of wine from the week and then have all of it on Friday or Saturday night! Alcohol is just sugar and useless calories. You can get all the polyphenols that are supposed to be in red wine, from other foods and dark chocolate. From my own personal experience and from other people's experience who have done our programme, it's hard to stick at just one small glass of wine! You will feel much better without it anyway.

The following is further example of our daily menu for the next four weeks.

Breakfast	20 grams mixed nuts.
	50 grams sheep's yoghurt.
Lunch	80 grams leftover roast lamb.
	Mixed salad of Chinese Leaves, celery, radishes, half an avocado and olives, dressed with olive oil.
Dinner	2 x roast chicken thighs.
	Sautéed cauliflower, onions, mushrooms, ginger and garlic, plus some Indian spices.

Remember, those veggies don't just need to be boiled or steamed. Roast them in the oven. Roasted chunks of red cabbage and roast brussels sprouts are fab, as is broccoli and cauliflower. Roast cauliflower and cumin seeds are great with curries. Use thinly sliced white cabbage for tagliatelle or spaghetti. You can cook it in a big bowl in the microwave. Just splash the sliced cabbage with olive oil, salt, pepper and microwave on full for about ten minutes, stirring halfway through cooking. Add a knob of butter at the end and some dried oregano. It's really tasty. Ok it's not pasta, but it does fill you up and it's great for your gut's good bacteria!

Chapter 10:
Six week review

So that's your first six weeks done. If you feel like we felt after six weeks, I don't need to write anything further! You'll know exactly what we mean.

However, I realise that there will be some of you who aren't quite there yet and have some more weight to lose, like we did at that stage, or have fallen off the plan slightly. If you are either of these, don't panic. Just stay with it. You'll not be far away. You should all be a good few pounds lighter by now, have more energy and should have started feeling a lot better about yourselves.

If you have reached the weight you want to be and have enjoyed the last six weeks way of eating, carry on with what you are doing now but increase your resistant starches. That is sweet potatoes and parsnips. You can also add in additional fruit, but keep an eye on your weight. If it starts to creep up again, cut out the fruit, and resistant starches.

Start experimenting with some of the baking recipes in this book. Some of the cakes and the fruit Bakewell pudding are lovely. You would not believe they don't have traditional flours in them. Don't be tempted to use proper sugar in any of your desserts. Steer clear of sugar completely and forever!

If you still have plenty of weight to lose, just stick to what you've been eating for the past four weeks. We stuck with it strictly for nine months, until we lost the weight we wanted. We still don't actually move very far away from

the same food now. We just experiment with different fruit and veg, but haven't gone back to bread, rice or pasta at all. We don't feel the need to now and I'm sure we won't be going back there again. We've got as much, if not more, energy now without them and for us, they just pile on the pounds, because it's hard to know when to stop eating them.

A funny story crops up here about bread, well toast actually.

We were travelling, either to or from, a caravan holiday and we pulled into a Little Chef somewhere on the A1 for breakfast. They were advertising that you could have as much tea/coffee and toast as you could eat and drink with every full breakfast you ordered. Well there was Julie, our two boys and myself. We all ordered full breakfasts and needless to say, the staff had their work cut out supplying us four with toast, butter and marmalade as well as coffee. Several loaves later we headed back up the AI. The only thing we were full of, was chat about what was for tea later that day!

Incidentally, we discovered that the Little Chef offer had finished, again whilst travelling on the AI, a short time later. I'm sure it wasn't anything to do with us, but a mere coincidence!

Chapter 11:
Exercise - get moving!

Exercise

At this point I need to mention the subject of exercise. Is it necessary or just another topic that has been confused by the 'experts'?

Well the answer is yes, to both questions but it's to what extent you need to actually exercise.

For both of us, it's been an important part of our lives for a long time. Even before we met each other. Julie has always been a very keen swimmer and regularly competed to a national level in her younger years with a deal of success. I have been a fan of the gym and weight/strength training since my late teens and at one time competed in bodybuilding competitions. We still partake in our chosen sports and fitness regimes, however, these days they overlap each other and I now swim fairly regularly and Julie comes to the gym with me.

Some years ago the 'experts' claimed that weight loss was achievable through a ratio of 70% training and 30% diet. That's now changed to about 60% training and 40% diet. I would argue that it's actually about 30% training and 70% diet. Completely the opposite way around to what it was.

This is our opinion, based on our experience of having done both over the years. We trained and still train, really quite intensively and it's only the last eighteen months, whilst on our current eating plan, that we have achieved the results we want. As I've mentioned before, it really felt that we were flogging a dead horse sometimes.

Compared to what we used to eat, we now eat very little protein, just the 200 grams per day of animal proteins and some additional nuts. Some days we don't eat animal protein at all and only have nuts and hemp seed. We don't have any additional protein supplements in the form of shakes etc. You don't need them. We're also as strong now, as we were two years ago when we were carrying all that weight around. We're loads fitter as well.

Our exercise consists of the following:

Gym

We split our bodies into two. One day we train legs, shoulders and biceps. The next day we train chest, back and triceps. We train stomachs just about every day and do approximately 20 mins of cardio, either on the treadmill or cross trainer.

If you aren't a regular user of the gym, then find your local one and seek advice from someone there before embarking on anything you do. Always start off slowly and do full body workouts first. Do weights/resistance type exercises over any type of cardio first. Resistance exercises are the ones that burn the fat. Cardio doesn't, unless you get into the realms of long distance type training. This is especially true if you are over 45 years old. As you get older, resistance exercises become even more important. You will not become muscle bound or build massive muscles, contrary to what you might believe or have been told in the past. This includes both males and females.

Swimming

Swimming is excellent as it is the only exercise that works every muscle in your body, whether you are male or female. It is one of the kindest exercises as the water supports your body, so it does not matter if you are able bodied,

disabled or even injured! As with any new exercise regime, you will need to start off slowly.

ALWAYS seek advise from your local pool, regarding a refresher course or lessons, to enable you to get your confidence back in the water. But if you prefer, go with a good friend who swims regularly, if you are feeling nervous or unsure.

The main thing is to ENJOY it, have FUN - IT WILL BE DOING YOUR BODY/MIND A WORLD OF GOOD!

Julie's Swimming

I have swum all my life, since the age of 12, at all different levels, including competitions. However nowadays I regularly swim twice a week usually between 1 - 1½ hours per session. I cover between 1 - 2 miles per session depending on how busy the pool is.

Martin's Swimming

Unless we are on our holidays, Martin's swimming is sporadic! In a 1-hour session, he usually does between 30 - 40 lengths, again depending on how busy the pool is.

To be honest Martin's preference is the gym,

Note

Never ever swim with sickness, diarrhoea or any other stomach problem, if in doubt always consult a medical expert. Never swim on a full stomach or under the influence of alcohol.

We appreciate that exercise is really not everybody's thing. We also realise that for some, because of a disability or even their current size, exercise is very difficult.

If you're just one of those people who have never or seldom exercised before, well now is the time to start. We're not suggesting that you go out and buy a gym membership or start training for the next Olympics or anything like that. Just start off slowly.

Start walking wherever and whenever possible. Attempt to build up to 10,000 steps a day slowly. Most phones these days have a step counter on them or just download one of the apps.

Some of our friends and neighbours had asked us what we were doing when it became obvious we were losing weight. They actually laughed at our training programmes and totally refused to have anything to do with our ideas. However we explained about just getting active and moving. We suggested starting walking a bit more regularly. Guess what? They can be seen most days walking round the block. Even during bad weather.

For those who are disabled in any way, always seek advice before starting any exercise. There is plenty of advice available from your local doctors about places that do classes for the disabled etc. More importantly though: don't be put off by your disability or size.

There is also loads of advice on the Internet about what you can do in the privacy of your own home if that's best for you.

The message here is, though, everybody needs to do something, no matter how much. Get to know what you enjoy and what your limitations are, but GET ACTIVE!

The thing about exercise is, it's a habit-forming activity. A good habit at that. It's also quite addictive due to the hormones your body releases during and after exercise. It makes you feel good both mentally and physically. Just don't go at it like a bull at a gate. Slowly does it at first!!

Chapter 12:
Eating out, dinner parties and holidays

Eating out and dinner parties

Eating out and dinner parties have been, and continue to be, a slight 'fly in the ointment'. Firstly dinner parties. We've found that it's always easier to host a dinner party rather than be a dinner party guest. When we host a dinner party we make and give our guests food that we now eat everyday. We do initially get a few turned up noses when they realise what they are going to eat, but that attitude, in the main, changes when they have actually eaten it.

An example of what we would serve is as follows:

Starter	Either soup or guacamole, with some veggie crudités.
Main Course	Either a piece of nicely roasted meat with loads of roasted veggies from the yes list or the vegetable cottage pie and a big mixed salad.
Dessert	No-bake cheesecake or the apple Bakewell pudding, both are from our recipes. Serve with double cream, crème fraiche or Greek yogurt.
Cheese and coffee	Flaxseed crackers and some nice local cheeses. You only need a little cheese!

This is just an example of what we have served and everyone, bar none, has been really surprised and commented that they didn't think we ate like that, or as much as that.

Curries with roasted cauliflower and onions are also good. You can always cook a bit of rice for your guests, so long as you don't eat it. Even quicker, buy some of that pre-cooked rice and just heat it up in the microwave!

Talking of microwaves, everything in our recipes can be cooked beforehand either heated up in the oven or microwave when your guests arrive, apart from salads. The cottage pie re-heats beautifully!

Look through the recipes in this book and make up your own menu. You will be surprised how much other people will enjoy your new food.

Being a guest at someone's house is a little more difficult because there is always a fear you may offend them by telling them what you can and can't eat. Don't be afraid to give them a ring beforehand and explain how well you're doing and how you really don't want to stall your success by over indulging on food you shouldn't be eating. Better to do it beforehand than on the night. We just tell people that we don't eat carbs such as rice, pasta, potatoes, bread, pastry and normal puddings. We always offer to take something with us such as a dessert or a big salad.

If you're going to a party or barbecue and the food is going to be a help yourself buffet style affair, well that makes life a lot easier. We tend to have our meal before we go and then just put some food on a plate and maybe just eat some salad and push the rest around our plates. Nobody notices or realises what you're doing. It makes life a lot easier for you. Also, take your own bottle of sparkling water, add a slice of lemon, plus ice and pretend it's a gin and tonic.

Eating out is slightly less problematic. If we know where we are going, we will ring before we get there and ask if they can make us a salad with either fish or meat. We normally tell them we're on a special diet and generally they are accommodating. If they aren't, we generally don't bother going.

Indian restaurants always seem to be easier.

We just have a tandoori chicken starter with some salad, a main course each and a couple of vegetable dishes like okra, mushroom, cauliflower or spinach. Just make sure it hasn't got potatoes or rice in them. Also no naan, other breads or poppadums. The pickle tray is also off limits, except for the yogurt and mint sauce.

Whether eating out or eating with friends at their home or yours you will be tempted to eat something you shouldn't. Don't be surprised if you end up actually gorging yourselves with what you shouldn't be eating and then afterwards feel terrible and very guilty.

We've been there and suffered the consequences. It's always difficult to get back on the straight and narrow afterwards. Best to just say no right from the start. Next day you'll be glad you did.

We can honestly say we don't, or rarely miss, the food we used to eat. Without exception. That includes cakes, sweets and milk chocolate. We've found that our sweet tooth has completely gone now and the berries we now eat are really sweet. We've discovered that lemons/limes aren't sour anymore and we add them just peeled and chopped to salads that we have with fish.

Holidays

The time will come when it's time for holidays. We realise that holidays can't be put off, especially if you have a family, or if it's just you and your partner. Don't panic. You just need to remember that you are not on a temporary quick fix diet, but living a new lifestyle completely, that isn't about to just change. You just need to stick to the same foods you are currently eating. Remember to watch the booze. Yes I know you're on your hols, but keep in the back of your mind how good you are feeling now.

Don't jeopardise all the success you are now enjoying, for that extra alcoholic drink or plate of chips!

We've been on several holidays abroad since we started our journey and apart from a couple of hiccups, we actually came back home having lost at least a couple of pounds. This has including eating out as well as preparing and cooking our own food. This has, of course, meant going self-catering so we have been in control of what we have bought and eaten.

If you do go 'all inclusive', concentrate on the salads, veggies, fish and meat. Avoid the sauces and steer clear of the puddings and cakes. Be careful of having too much fresh fruit, remember they are full of hidden sugars!

It's well worth the effort in the long run.

Chapter 13:
People's attitudes and opinions

We have been completely taken aback by the change in attitudes and opinions of people, before, during and after our weight loss: perhaps naively.

When we were fat and really quite unhappy about the fact, we seemed to have far more friends and acquaintances than we have now. We were generally accepted by everyone and had a good social life. Almost all our friends and families have changed their attitudes towards us, some for the better, some not. We feel slightly less accepted by some people and a few 'friends' have actually gone out of their way to be just unfriendly and awkward with us.

We think, in the main, that this is just jealousy. A lot of people we know or knew, are always on some kind of diet, like we were, and are still that way now, despite quizzing us about what and how we were achieving our success.

I realise that there is a danger that we have become slightly over enthusiastic about our success and really want to tell the world how healthy, different and fabulous we feel now. So we try to temper that attitude and unless someone wants to seriously talk to us about what we've done, we just gloss over the details if we are at a social event. However we offer to meet that person if they are genuinely interested at a later date, convenient to all of us, to answer and discuss any questions or queries they may have.

Remember this programme and subsequent success is for you and you alone. Don't let other people's opinions and negativity stop you doing what you know you can achieve and carry on achieving for the rest of your lives.

Chapter 14:
Time to start eating properly

Oven conversions

Gas	Fahrenheit	Celsius	Fan
1	275	140	120
2	300	150	130
3	325	170	150
4	350	180	160
5	375	190	170
6	400	200	180
7	425	220	200
8	450	230	210
9	475	240	220

BREAKFASTS

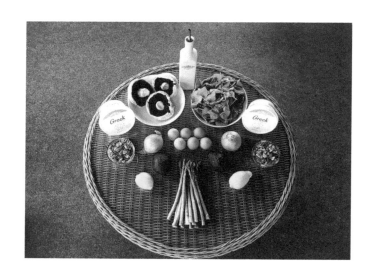

Green Smoothie

Serves 2

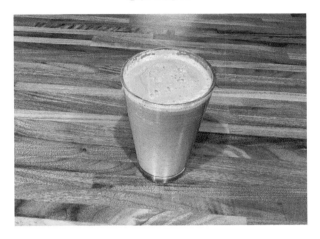

INGREDIENTS

250 ml hemp milk or unsweetened almond milk or water
½ ripe avocado, stoned, peeled and roughly chopped
1 medium carrot, roughly chopped
3 - 4 florets of broccoli
Handful of fresh mint leaves, chopped
Juice of a lemon
3 - 4 frozen balls of spinach
Salt and pepper to taste

METHOD

Place ingredients as above in that order into a blender.
Blend on full speed / power until smooth. You will probably have to let the smoothie down with water, so it's a looser consistency.
Pour into a glass and drink.
Any remaining smoothie put into a drinks container used for making protein shakes and refrigerate, remember to shake well before drinking.

Greek Yogurt with Mixed Toasted Nuts

Serves 2

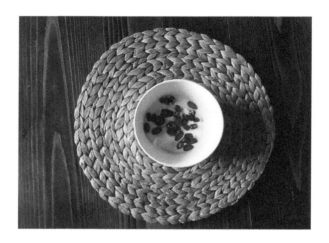

INGREDIENTS

2 dessertspoons Greek, goats or sheeps yogurt of your choice
Toasted mixed nuts, (we use brazils, pecans, walnuts, almonds)

METHOD

Prepare your choice of nuts first, by toasting them in hot oven, making sure you
don't burn them.
Place your yogurt into a dish, then place your required amount of nuts on top.
Serve and enjoy.

NOTE:

We tend to toast lots of nuts at one time, let them cool, store them in an airtight
container until we need them. A good guide we have found is: ladies 30 grams,
gentlemen 50 grams.

Mushroom and Onion Frittata

Serves 2

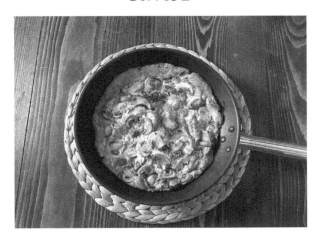

INGREDIENTS

4 large eggs (free range or organic if possible)
6 - 8 thinly sliced mushrooms
I medium thinly sliced onion
I teaspoon dried oregano
I tablespoon olive oil
Salt and pepper to taste

METHOD

Prepare all your ingredients.
Beat the eggs with a tablespoon of water or milk, season with a pinch of salt, pepper and oregano.
Heat oil on a medium heat in a 28 cm non-stick frying pan. When oil is hot, fry onion until soft and slightly browned.
Add mushrooms and continue frying until they turn slightly brown.
Give the beaten egg mixture a further quick whisk/beat then add to your frying pan.

Using a spatula gently stir egg away from the pan edges.

Then leave mixture for approximately a minute, so it forms a large pancake, but it is still soft and a bit runny on top.

Remove from the heat!

Place under a hot grill, continue to cook/grill until the frittata swells up, is golden brown, and all the egg is cooked.

Remove from under the grill, allow to cool for a couple of minutes, then turn out the Frittata onto a chopping board, cut into pizza style wedges.

Serve with a big bowl of mixed salad.

This is beautiful cold the next day and again can be served with a big bowl of mixed salad.

Grilled Field Mushrooms
with Homemade Pesto Sauce
Serves 2

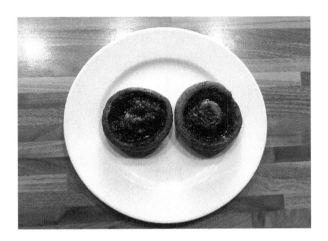

INGREDIENTS
1 - 2 field mushrooms per person depending on their size
1 - 2 teaspoons of pesto sauce per mushroom depending on taste
1 - 2 teaspoons refined olive oil
Salt and pepper to taste

METHOD
Pre heat the grill to HOT.
Put your mushrooms upside down into grill pan, drizzle with oil, salt and pepper.
Place grill pan under preheated grill, until mushrooms are almost cooked,
remove from grill.
Spread pesto sauce on top of each mushroom.
Return to hot grill and continue grilling until the pesto turns slightly brown.
Serve and enjoy.

NOTE

Homemade pesto sauce recipe can be found in 'Side dishes and Accompaniments' section of this book.

If using bought pesto sauce CHECK label for hidden sugars, non-compliant oil e.g. vegetable or rape seed oils.

Egg and Spinach Gratin
Serves 2

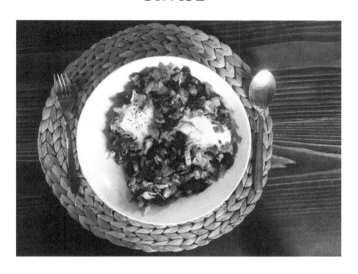

INGREDIENTS

l full 300 grams bag of washed baby spinach leaves
l medium thinly sliced onion
2 cloves of garlic peeled, crushed and finely chopped
8 medium mushrooms thinly sliced
l medium carrot thinly sliced into batons
4 large eggs
l teaspoon dried oregano
Salt and pepper to taste
Pinch of chilli powder to sprinkle/dust each egg
2 tablespoons refined olive oil
25 grams blue/strong cheddar/or grated Parmesan cheese

METHOD

Prepare your ingredients, then preheat the grill to FULL.

Heat olive oil in a frying pan/sauté pan on a medium heat till the oil is hot, add in carrot, onion and fry until just starting to turn golden brown, but not burnt, approximately 5 minutes.

Next add in garlic, stir into carrot and onion.

Add in mushrooms, fry everything until all is soft but not mushy.

Empty full bag of spinach in next, allow it to wilt down completely. (A big bag of spinach will wilt down quite considerably, far more than you expect.)

Add in salt, pepper and herbs.

Make 4 wells into your softened vegetables, then crack one egg into each of the wells. Sprinkle/dust each egg with a little chilli powder (too much will make it too hot), then sprinkle on top the cheese of your choice.

Place your pan under the preheated hot grill, cook until the cheese has all melted and the eggs have just set.

Serve 2 eggs, plus half of the cooked vegetables per person.

We often serve it with a basic salad, if serving for lunch or dinner. Enjoy.

LUNCHES

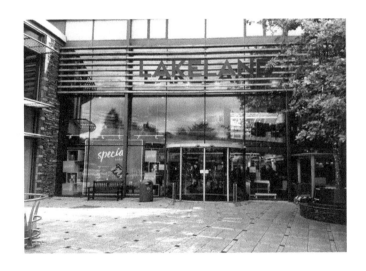

Basic Salad with Leftover Chicken

Serves 2

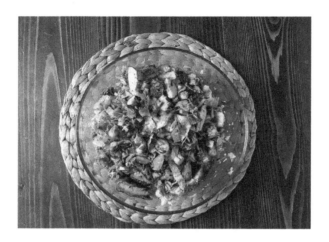

INGREDIENTS

Basic Salad ingredients can be found in 'Side Dishes and Accompaniments' in this book

100 grams of cold cooked chicken or meat/fish of your choice

METHOD

Prepare your basic salad as in 'Sides Dishes and Accompaniments' section of this book.

Slice up the leftover cooked cold meat of your choice and place into bowl with your prepared basic salad. Combine thoroughly. Serve and enjoy.

Tuna Salad

Serves 2

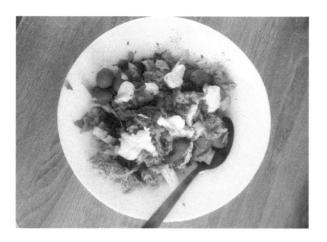

INGREDIENTS

1 tin tuna per person, (either in olive oil or water, drain it)
Romaine lettuce (or any of your choice)
3 - 4 thinly sliced radishes 2 sticks of celery, chopped
Avocado, peeled and chopped
3 raw mushrooms, sliced thinly
2 small raw carrots, chopped or grated
12 green or black olives pitted
2 teaspoons herbs provencal
2 dessertspoons of extra virgin olive oil
Salt and pepper to taste

METHOD

Prepare all your salad ingredients.

Toss them into a pasta bowl, including olives, avocado, olive oil, herbs, salt and pepper.

Add the drained tuna on top.

We serve it with 1 tablespoon of full fat Greek yogurt per person.

Enjoy.

Toasted Mixed Nuts/Hemp Seed Salad

Serves 2

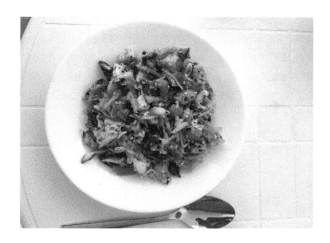

INGREDIENTS

60 grams mixed toasted nuts
25 grams toasted hemp seeds
4 romaine lettuce leaves sliced
2 radishes sliced
l large carrot grated
2 sticks celery chopped
l avocado peeled, stone removed and sliced
l inch red cabbage finely sliced
12 green or black pitted olives
l tablespoon sauerkraut
l teaspoon mixed herbs
l tablespoon extra virgin olive oil
Salt and pepper to taste

METHOD

Lightly toast the mixed nuts, we use almonds, pecans, walnuts, Brazil nuts, separately from the hemp seed, (as hemp seeds burn quickly).

Mix together the nuts and hemp seeds, leave them to cool completely.

Place all the remaining ingredients into a large bowl, mix really well.

Once the nuts and hemp seeds are cold, add to the large bowl of salad and mix thoroughly.

Serve and enjoy.

This is our favourite salad!

Pan Fried Salmon with Basic Salad

Serves 2

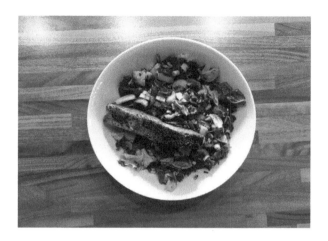

INGREDIENTS

2 x 100 grams piece of salmon (1 per person)
2 tablespoons refined olive oil
Salt and pepper to taste
Basic salad recipe can be found in 'Side Dishes and Accompaniments' section of this book.

METHOD

Prepare your basic salad.
Place the salmon on a plate and drizzle all over with refined olive oil and sprinkle all over with salt and pepper.
Heat a frying pan over a low - medium heat and place salmon skin side down in pan. Fry until skin turns crispy or golden brown about 4 minutes. Then turn salmon and fry on all other sides for about 2 minutes per side.
Serve with your prepared basic salad.

Crudités
Serves 2

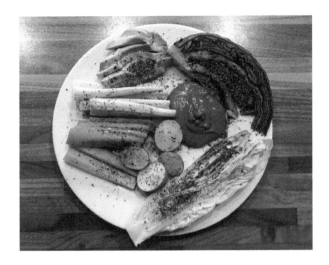

INGREDIENTS
1 avocado, peeled, stoned and sliced (we use a ½ per person)
¼ romaine lettuce, leave whole including the stalk (per person)
½ inch slice of red cabbage, including the stalk (per person)
1 stick celery, cut into batons (per person)
1 medium carrot, cut into batons (per person)
2 medium radishes, cut into ½ (per person)
1 - 2 tablespoons extra virgin olive oil
1 - 2 teaspoons mixed herbs or your favourite choice of herbs
Salt and pepper to taste

METHOD
Prepare your chosen vegetables as above.
Arrange on serving plate, add the oil, herbs salt and pepper to taste.
Serve and enjoy.

NOTE
This can be used as:
A quick lunch,
A starter, or
A snack

Our photo shows it with homemade nut butter - delicious!

It is great to experiment with different vegetables and herbs of your choice, until you find your favourite one. We use the same amounts per person so this recipe can be made for more people.

Cheesy Feta Vegetables

Serves 2

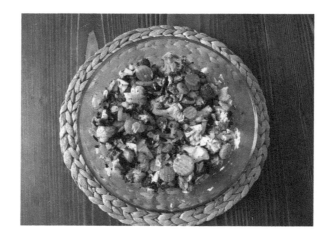

INGREDIENTS

1 large onion, finely sliced

6 mushrooms, finely sliced

1 clove garlic, peeled and crushed

¼ of large white cabbage, finely sliced

250 grams frozen vegetables (we use cauliflower, broccoli,)

250 grams frozen sprouts (optional)

4 balls frozen spinach

250 grams Greek feta cheese, chopped into cubes

2 tablespoons refined olive oil

2 teaspoons mixed herbs

Salt and pepper to taste

METHOD

Put prepared cabbage into a large microwave bowl, place in microwave, on full power for 5 minutes until soft.

Add rest of frozen vegetables to cabbage, return to the microwave, cook them on full power for approximately 10 minutes more or until soft.

Whilst vegetables are in the microwave cooking, fry the prepared onions, mushrooms, and garlic in 1 tablespoon of olive oil until they are all soft.

Chop the feta cheese into cubes.

When everything is cooked mix them together.

Add the remaining tablespoon of olive oil, mixed herbs, salt and pepper, return the bowl into the microwave, on full power for 2 - 3 minutes more, or until feta cheese has softened. This recipe is great for a quick tea on holiday.

Broccoli Soup

Serves 2

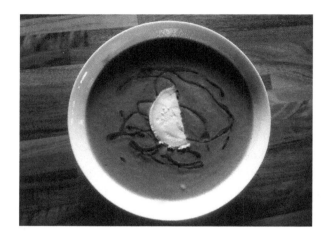

INGREDIENTS

2 heads of broccoli, chop into small florets
1 large onion, peeled and thinly sliced
½ inch piece of fresh ginger, peeled and roughly chopped
1 clove garlic, peeled, grated or smashed
1 teaspoon thyme or oregano
1 tablespoon refined olive oil
1 - 1½ litres of water
Salt and pepper to taste

METHOD

Place oil into a large pan, put on medium heat, and fry onion, garlic and ginger until soft. Then add water, broccoli, salt, pepper plus herbs of your choice, bring everything to the boil, then simmer until soft.
Blend with a stick blender, add extra water if soup is too thick. Serve and enjoy.

VARIATIONS

We add per person:

20 grams slice of goats cheese <u>or</u>

Half an avocado sliced <u>or</u>

50 grams toasted flaked almonds, sprinkle on top <u>or</u>

30 grams toasted hemp seed, sprinkle on top <u>or</u>

25 grams grated parmesan cheese, sprinkle on top <u>or</u>

1 dessertspoon of soured cream, poured on top.

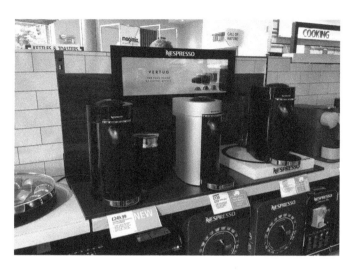

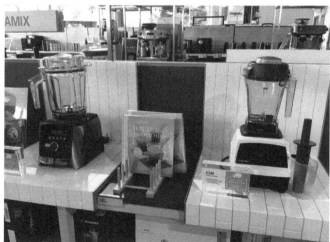

Kitchen accessories at Lakeland.

SNACKS

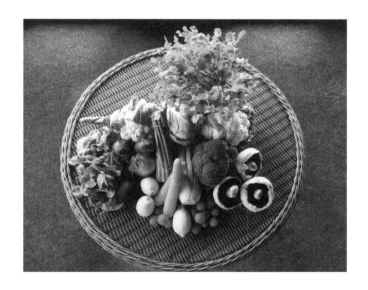

Flaxseed Crackers

Makes 30 - 35

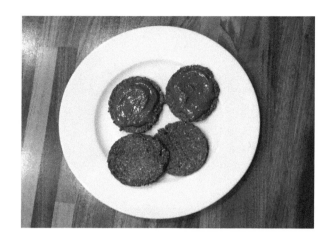

INGREDIENTS

4 large egg whites
20 grams stevia or sweetener of your choice
150 grams ground flaxseeds
150 grams ground almonds
Pinch of salt
Pinch of coarse ground black pepper

METHOD

Preheat the oven to 170 C, Fan 150 C, 325 F, Gas 3
You will need 2 baking trays lined with baking parchment.
Place egg whites and sweetener of your choice into a large bowl and using an
electric mixer, whisk together until they form stiff peaks.
Fold in flaxseeds, ground almonds, salt and black pepper, and combine all
ingredients until mixture forms a large dough ball.

Place dough ball in between 2 sheets of parchment paper, roll out dough until it is approximately 5 mm thick.

Remove top sheet of parchment, cut mixture into 5 cm rounds, gently re-roll any scraps. (Remember to replace top parchment sheet prior to rolling it again.)

Cut more crackers until all the dough has been used up.

Using a palette knife or spatula place rounds on prepared baking trays lined with non-stick baking liner, bake in preheated oven for 30 - 35 minutes or until golden brown.

Remove from oven, leave on baking trays for 5 minutes to cool allowing them to firm up, then transfer crackers onto cooling racks until they are completely cold.

Serve or store in an airtight container for up to 10 days if you can resist them!

VARIATIONS

You can replace 150 grams ground flaxseeds with 50 grams hemp seeds plus 100 grams ground flaxseeds

Both recipes are equally tasty.

SERVE

With goats or sheep cheese but remember to get it out of the fridge before you need it so it can reach room temperature. <u>OR</u>

Homemade Nut Butter (recipe can be found under 'Side Dishes and Accompaniments' section of this book).

Also, the thinner you make the crackers, the crispier they are but be aware they will not need as long in the oven. If you do make thinner ones you will make more than 30 - 35 crackers.

Guacamole

Serves 4

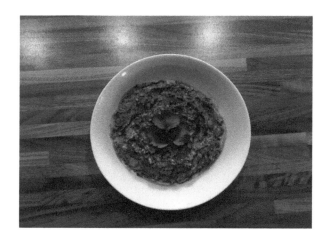

INGREDIENTS
1 ripe avocado, peeled, remove stone
1 tablespoon almond nut butter
¼ teaspoon chilli powder
Juice of 1 lime
2 spring onions, thinly sliced
Handful of chopped coriander (optional)
Salt and pepper to taste

METHOD
Place your prepared avocado into a dish, mash with a fork until smooth. Mix in almond nut butter, until smooth.

Add in chilli, lime juice, spring onions, (coriander if using) plus salt and pepper, combine all ingredients thoroughly.

Drizzle over the top with extra virgin olive oil.

98

Serve with cos or romaine lettuce leaves, or celery and carrot sticks or wedges of red/white cabbage.

NOTE
Homemade Nut Butter recipes can be found under 'Side Dishes and Accompaniments' in this book.

Red or White Cabbage Leaves with Mixed Toasted Nuts - (Our Sandwiches)

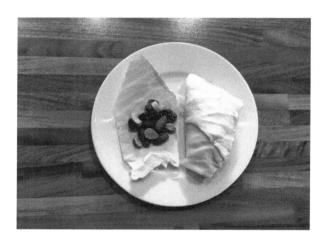

INGREDIENTS

Select your choice of cabbage leaves either red or white, remove from cabbage (we usually do 2 leaves per person)

20 grams mixed toasted nuts (we use pecan, walnuts, almonds, brazil)

METHOD

Prepare the nuts.

Select your choice of cabbage, remove 2 leaves per person, we leave the tender bit of the stalk in.

Place a mixture of prepared nuts onto the middle of each leaf, then fold the leaves up as in the picture above.

Ready made 'sandwiches' which we find are more filling than bread and much healthier for you.

Good for pack ups.

Lettuce Leaves with Nut Butter (Our Sandwiches)

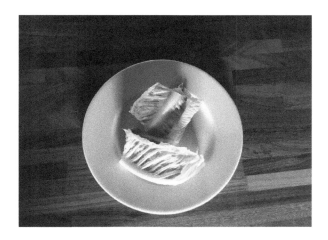

INGREDIENTS

Romaine or cos lettuce leaves, (we use 2 leaves per person)
Home made Nut butter, recipe can be found in 'Side Dishes and
Accompaniments' section of this book.
Salt and pepper to taste

METHOD

Make sure you have made your nut butter in advance.
Select the lettuce of your choice, remove two leaves per person.
Spread 2 teaspoons of nut butter onto each leaf, spreading it out down the
centre.
Fold the leaves as in the photo above.
We find these very filling and we seriously don't miss bread!
Can be prepared in advance for pack ups.

DINNERS

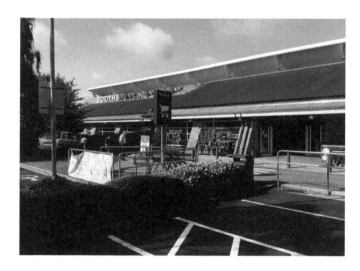

Booths supermarket, our local!

Vegetable Cottage Pie

Serves 4
Freezes well

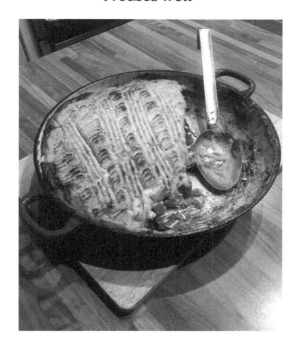

INGREDIENTS

500 grams sprouts, trimmed and cut in half (if in season) or use instead ⅓ medium white cabbage, cut into ½ inch pieces

I large onion, thinly sliced

I - 2 cloves garlic peeled, chopped, finely sliced

2 medium carrots, finely diced

¼ medium swede, peeled cut into small cubes/pieces or use instead 2 medium parsnips, cut into ½ inch cubes

2 tablespoons refined olive oil

6 - 8 mushrooms, thinly sliced
2 tablespoons water or white wine
1 tablespoon tomato purée
Juice of fresh lemon
200 grams block feta cheese, cut into 1-inch cubes/pieces
1 dessertspoon dried thyme
1 dessertspoon fennel seeds
Salt and pepper to taste
1 portion of homemade cauliflower mash

HOMEMADE CAULIFLOWER MASH RECIPE
Can be found in the 'Side Dishes and Accompaniments' section of this book.

METHOD
Prepare all your ingredients.
Heat oil in a shallow casserole dish that has a lid.
When the oil is hot, add the fennel seeds, let them sizzle for a minute, now add in onion, carrot, swede, celery and fry gently over a medium heat for approximately 5 minutes until they start to soften.
Add sprouts, parsnips if using to pan and stir-fry for a further 2 minutes, then add mushrooms, garlic, and fry for 2 more minutes.
Stir in the tomato purée, keep frying for another 2 minutes.
Now add in water or white wine, plus dried herbs, salt and pepper.
Place the lid onto the dish, simmer for approximately 10 -15 minutes on a low heat, until all vegetables are soft, cooked, and there is very little liquid left.
Let all vegetables go cold in the dish, then dot with the feta cheese cubes, evenly around the vegetables in the dish.
Spoon the prepared cauliflower mash on top of the dish that contains your cooked vegetables/feta cheese cubes.

Spread out evenly with a spatula so all the vegetables/feta cheese is covered.
Run a fork over the surface of cauliflower mash so it forms a criss-cross pattern
on the top, i.e. #
If serving straight away, place in a preheated oven, 200 C, Fan 180 C, 400 F, Gas
6, bake for approximately 45 - 50 minutes, the top should be golden and slightly
crisp.

VARIATION

Prior to cooking, sprinkle 50 grams, grated Parmesan cheese on top of
cauliflower mash - which gives you an even crispier topping.
Serve by itself or with a side salad.

NOTE

Once pie is ready, it can be left till needed.
Place into a preheated oven 200 C, Fan 180 C, 400 F, Gas 6, bake for
approximately 45-50 minutes or until the top is golden brown.

Cabbage Tagliatelle
Serves 2

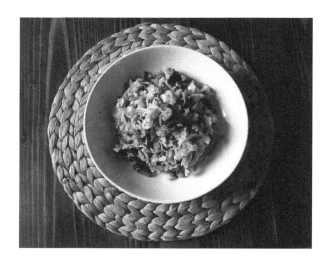

INGREDIENTS

⅔ of large thinly sliced white cabbage

1 large finely sliced onion

1 clove garlic, peeled and crushed

100 grams sliced mushrooms

1 tablespoon refined olive oil

Knob of butter

1 teaspoon mixed herbs

100 grams smoked bacon chopped into small pieces

60 grams smoked grated cheese or

60 grams cream cheese

Salt and pepper to taste

METHOD

Steam all the thinly sliced cabbage, until soft. This can be cooked on full power in microwave, or by steaming. Fry onion, bacon, and garlic in olive oil until soft. Add mushrooms, mixed herbs, continue frying until soft.

Next add cheese and mix in until cheese has melted and made a sauce. Place steamed cabbage in large bowl and add all the remaining ingredients, mixing thoroughly. Serve and enjoy.

Roasted Belly Pork Slices
with Sauté Vegetables

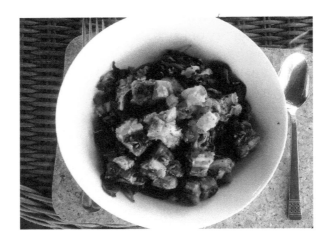

INGREDIENTS

FOR PORK
   1 belly pork slice (approx. 100 grams cooked) per person
   1 teaspoon fennel seeds
   1 teaspoon mixed herbs
   Salt and pepper to taste

FOR SAUTÉ VEGETABLES
   ½ medium red cabbage plus ½ medium Savoy cabbage, thinly sliced
   150 grams mushrooms, thinly sliced
   1 medium onion, thinly sliced
   1 clove garlic, peeled and crushed
   1 teaspoon cumin seeds
   1 tablespoon balsamic vinegar

1 tablespoon olive oil
2 handfuls pre-washed baby spinach leaves
Salt and pepper to taste

METHOD

FOR PORK

Score the belly pork rind/fat crossways, sprinkle with fennel seeds, salt, pepper and herbs.
Place in hot oven, 200 C, Fan 180 C, 400 F, Gas mark 6, for 1½ hours until cooked, and the belly pork rind/fat is nice and crispy.

FOR SAUTÉ VEGETABLES

Fry onion, cumin seeds in olive oil until soft and slightly brown on the edges.
Add red cabbage and fry until slightly brown on the edges.
Add mushrooms, garlic, herbs, Savoy cabbage, and continue to stir-fry until vegetables are soft.
Add spinach leaves, balsamic vinegar and keep stirring until all the liquid has thickened.

TO SERVE

Chop belly pork slices into bite size pieces and scatter on top of the vegetables.
Enjoy.

Slow Roasted Lamb with Rosemary and Roast Vegetables
Serves 2 - 4

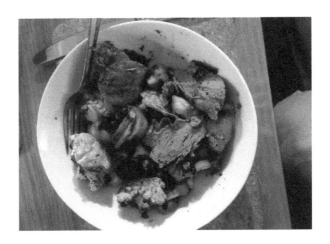

INGREDIENTS

Leg or Shoulder of Lamb (we prefer shoulder)

1 teaspoon dried rosemary or a couple of sprigs of fresh rosemary

1 medium head of cauliflower, cut into small florets, stalks as well

12 shallots (depends on size)

⅓ of red cabbage, cut into chunks

100 grams thinly sliced mushrooms

1 clove of garlic, peeled and cut into slivers

1 clove of garlic, peeled but left whole

1½ inch of peeled fresh ginger, finely chopped

1 teaspoon madras curry powder

1 teaspoon cumin seeds

2 tablespoons refined olive oil

Salt and pepper to taste

METHOD

FOR THE LAMB

Make slits in the lamb with a sharp small knife, fill the slits with slivers of one of the cloves of garlic.

Sprinkle lamb with rosemary, salt and pepper.

Place in a roasting tray in a preheated oven 170 C, Fan 150, 325 F, gas 3, for approximately 2 hours or until the lamb is very tender/falling apart.

FOR THE VEGETABLES

Peel shallots, leave whole, put in another roasting tray, with some of the oil, make sure the shallots are coated with oil, place in oven, underneath the shelf below the lamb, turn the oven up to 200 C, Fan 180, 400 F, gas 6.

Prepare remaining vegetables, then add to roasting tray which has the shallots in together with the rest of the oil, curry powder, cumin seeds, the other clove of garlic which is left whole, salt and pepper. Mix together, making sure they are all equally covered with the oil.

Roast for approximately 45 minutes, still at 200 C, Fan 180, 400 F, gas 6, until all the vegetables are cooked and slightly brown.

Serve and enjoy.

Basic Chicken Curry
Serves 2

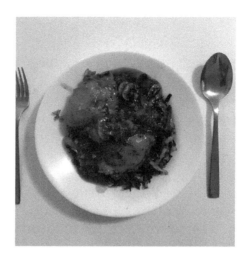

INGREDIENTS

4 chicken thighs skinned (2 each)
1 large onion, sliced
2 cloves garlic, crushed
1 inch square fresh ginger, peeled and crushed
75 grams sliced mushrooms
1 tin 400 grams chopped tomatoes
1 dessertspoon madras curry powder
2 tablespoons refined olive oil
Salt and pepper to taste

METHOD

Place oil in a frying pan, on a medium heat, when it is hot, add in the sliced onion and fry until soft and slightly brown. Add in crushed garlic, ginger to the

onions and fry for another minute. Then add curry powder in, stirring well.
Next add in chopped tomatoes, fry gently on a low heat for approx. 5 mins or
until liquid reduces.
Lastly add chicken, mushrooms, plus 400 ml water, simmer on a low heat for 45
mins approximately. Remember to place a lid on top of your pan.
Serve and enjoy.

You can swap 2 chicken thighs for 1 chicken breast sliced, per person. Remember
to cook it for 35 mins not 45 mins. There will be enough curry sauce in this
recipe for 4 people.

NOTE
We use either a sauté pan or a deep frying pan with a lid for this recipe.

Roast Chicken Tray Bake
Serves 2

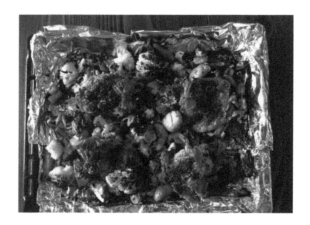

INGREDIENTS

4 chicken thighs, leave bone in and skin on, 2 per person, approx. 100 grams each

1 medium cauliflower, cut into florets, include stalks cut into 1 inch pieces

½ medium red cabbage, cut into 4, then cut each piece again into 4 pieces

2 - 3 medium onions, peeled, cut each one into 8 wedges

1 head of broccoli, cut into florets include stalks cut into 1 inch pieces

4 cloves of garlic, left whole with skins on

Refined olive oil as much as you need, so tray bake does not dry out

1 teaspoon dried thyme

1 teaspoon dried rosemary

1 teaspoon dried oregano

Salt and pepper to taste

NOTE

2 sweet potatoes can be added, but leave skin on and cut into 1 inch chunks. Omit these if you are just starting on the programme or you are desperate to reach your next target weight!

METHOD

Preheat oven to 200 C, Fan 180 C, 400 F, Gas 6.

Prepare all your ingredients as above.

If you are pushed for time or if you want to speed this up follow this method:

Place chicken thighs on a large roasting tray, sprinkle with salt, pepper and place uncovered, on middle shelf in preheated oven.

Place onion wedges onto a microwaveable plate. Drizzle with a little oil and microwave on full for 4 - 5 minutes until they are soft. Add softened onion to tray with chicken and return to oven.

Do the same with the red cabbage and add it to tray with chicken and onion.

At this point add all the other ingredients except the garlic, covering them liberally with olive oil. Sprinkle over herbs of your choice, plus salt and pepper.

Mix all ingredients around in the roasting tray until everything is coated in the oil.

Return to oven for a further 45 minutes.

Remove from oven and poke the cloves of garlic in between the vegetables and chicken.

Place back into the oven for a further 20 minutes or until garlic is soft, your vegetables are nicely browned and roasted.

Serve in big soup/pasta bowls.

Don't forget to include any of the oil/juices from the roasting tray. Enjoy.

Pepper Fry
Serves 4

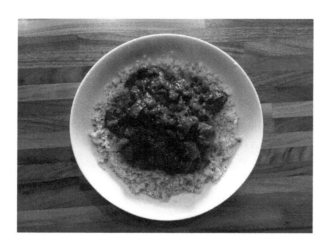

INGREDIENTS

1 kg shin beef (works best) or stewing beef, cut into 1½ inch cubes
1 x 400 grams tin chopped tomatoes
2 medium onions, thinly sliced
1½ inch square fresh ginger peeled and finely chopped
½ teaspoon turmeric
2 teaspoons coarse ground black pepper
2 tablespoons refined olive oil
Water
Salt to taste

METHOD

Prepare all your ingredients.
Heat oil in shallow casserole dish, without its lid, fry onions until slightly brown, add ginger and fry for 1 more minute.

Put in turmeric, coarse black pepper, stir well, continue to fry for a further
1 minute. Now add the chopped tomatoes and fry until the liquid from the
tomatoes reduces and quite a thick paste has formed.
Fill empty tomato tin completely with water, add this to your dish with the meat
and stir well.
Cover casserole dish with its lid and simmer on a low heat for approximately 1½
- 2 hours.

This recipe can be started on your hob, then when you reach where you add
the meat and water, you can cover it with its lid and put it into a preheated oven
160 C, Fan 140 C, 320 F, Gas 3 for 2 hours, or until meat is tender.
When meat is cooked and tender by whichever method you have cooked it,
remove lid and return to hob. Continue to cook on a medium heat until sauce
thickens and you end up with the sauce slightly sticking to the bottom of the
pan as it starts to fry.
HENCE the name/title PEPPER FRY.

NOTE
. This recipe can also be done with:
 1 kg chicken - cook for 1 hour (we find it best to remove the chicken from the
 pan prior to reducing sauce. Then add back in when sauce has thickened to
 reheat)
 1 kg pork - cook for 1½ to 2 hours
 1 kg venison - cook for 1½ to 2 hours
 1 kg diced lamb - cook for 1½ to 2 hours

The method is the same as above, whichever meat you use.

Pork and Beef Burgers
Serves 2

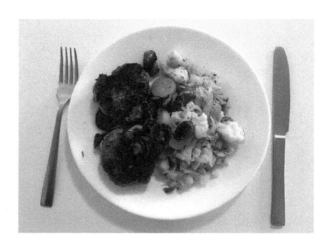

INGREDIENTS
  400 grams mixed pork and beef mince
  l teaspoon mixed herbs
  l teaspoon fennel seeds
  Salt and pepper to taste

METHOD
  Place pork and beef mince into a large bowl and mix thoroughly.
  Add mixed herbs, fennel seeds and ½ teaspoon coarse black pepper, mixing again
  thoroughly.
  Divide mixture into 4 and make burgers.
  Place onto a plate, cover with cling film, leave in the fridge to firm up. Sprinkle
  both sides of the burgers with salt, prior to cooking.
  Fry in frying pan, on a medium heat, with only the fat which the burgers release,
  for approximately 4 - 5 minutes each side or until firm to the touch.

  Serve with a large salad or an assortment of steamed vegetables.

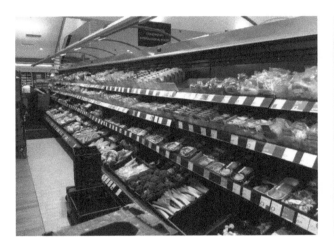
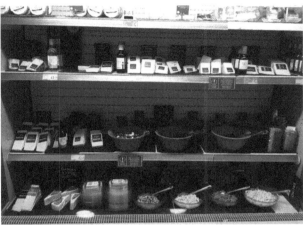
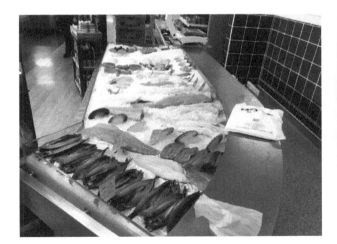
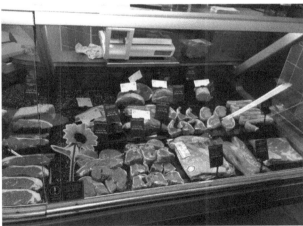

Local produce at Booths.

SIDE DISHES AND ACCOMPANIMENTS

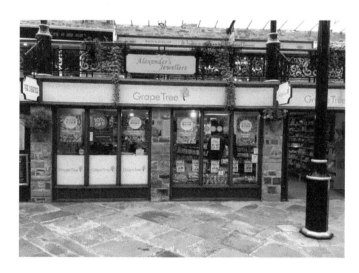

GrapeTree open for business.

Basic Salad

Serves 2-4

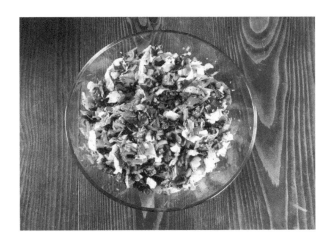

INGREDIENTS

6 leaves Romaine lettuce, finely sliced

4 - 6 radishes finely sliced, depends on their size

1 stick of celery, finely sliced

½ medium red onion, finely sliced

Small wedge of red cabbage, finely shredded

Small wedge of white cabbage, finely shredded

1 dessertspoon dried oregano

1 dessertspoon toasted milled flaxseeds (optional)

2 - 3 tablespoons extra virgin olive oil

6 - 12 pitted olives green or black

Salt and pepper to taste

Whole avocado, peeled and chopped into small cubes

METHOD

Prepare all your vegetables, place them into a large bowl, with herbs, flaxseeds if using, extra virgin olive oil, salt and pepper.

Mix thoroughly until all ingredients are combined. Serve straight away.

If you prepare this salad in advance, leave salt and oil out until just prior to serving, then mix them in thoroughly. Place in fridge, covered with cling film, (remember to get salad out of fridge, 30 minutes - 1 hour before needed so it reaches room temperature before serving). Serve and enjoy.

Red - White Cabbage Coleslaw/Salad

Serves 2

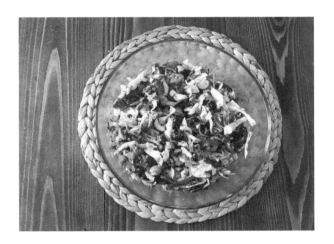

INGREDIENTS

¼ of a small white and red cabbage, sliced thinly

2 medium red onions, sliced thinly/shredded

2 raw carrots, grated or diced

2 sticks celery, chopped

3- 4 radishes, sliced/chopped

12 green or black pitted olives

1 avocado, peeled and chopped

1 dessertspoon mixed herbs

2 dessertspoons extra virgin olive oil

Salt and pepper to taste

METHOD

Prepare all your salad ingredients, chopped, sliced, or shredded and place into a large mixing bowl.

Add the olives, prepared avocado, herbs and olive oil. Mix ingredients thoroughly. Serve and enjoy.

We add, per person:
100 grams roasted chicken or
100 grams pan-fried salmon or
60 grams tinned tuna or
25 grams goats cheese or
30 grams mixed toasted nuts (ladies), 50 grams (men)

Vegetable Tray Bake
Serves 2

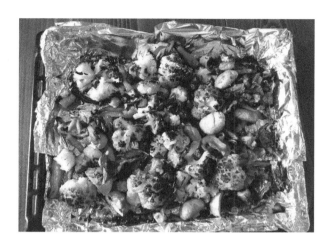

INGREDIENTS
1 medium cauliflower cut in florets, include stalks cut into 1 inch pieces
½ medium red cabbage cut into 4, then cut each piece into 4 again
2 - 3 medium onions, peeled then cut each one into 8 wedges
1 head of broccoli cut into florets, include stalks cut into 1 inch pieces
4 cloves garlic left whole with skins on
Refined olive oil, as much as you need, so tray bake does not dry out
1 teaspoon dried thyme
1 teaspoon dried rosemary
1 teaspoon dried oregano
Salt and pepper to taste

VARIATION
2 sweet potatoes can also be added, leave the skin on and cut into 1 inch chunks.
Omit these if you are just starting the programme or you are desperate to reach
your next target weight!

METHOD

Preheat your oven to 200 C, Fan 180 C, 400 F, Gas 6.

Prepare all your ingredients as above.

If you are pushed for time or if you want to speed this up, follow this method;

Place onion wedges onto microwave plate.

Drizzle with a little oil and microwave on full for 4 - 5 minutes until they are soft.

Add softened onion onto oven tray and place in oven on middle shelf.

Do the same with the red cabbage then add it to the tray with the onion.

At this point, add all the other ingredients except the garlic, covering them liberally with the olive oil.

Sprinkle over herbs of your choice, plus salt and pepper.

Mix everything around in the roasting tray until everything is coated in the oil.

Return to the oven for a further 45 minutes.

Remove from oven and poke the cloves of garlic in between the vegetables.

Return to the oven for a further 20 minutes or until garlic is soft and the vegetables are nicely browned and roasted.

Serve in big soup/pasta bowls.

Don't forget to include any of the oil/juices from the roasting tray.

NOTE

This is a vegetarian dish, but either nuts or cheese could also be added.

However, it can be used as a side dish for any meat, fish or poultry main dish.

Enjoy.

Basic Sauté Red and White Cabbage
Serves 2

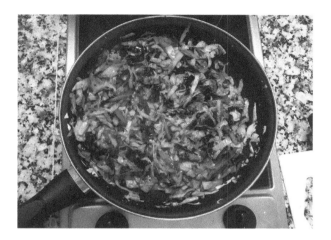

INGREDIENTS

  1 large carrot, thinly sliced into batons
  ½ inch slice of red cabbage, thinly sliced
  ½ inch slice of white cabbage, thinly sliced
  1 tablespoon of refined olive oil
  Good knob of butter
  1 teaspoon fennel seeds
  Salt and pepper to taste

METHOD

  Melt butter and oil in frying pan on a low heat.
  Add prepared red cabbage, carrot and sauté until soft, approximately 5 minutes.
  Now add in prepared white cabbage, continue to sauté until all veg is soft.
  Salt and pepper to taste.

VARIATIONS

This recipe can be altered by using any vegetables that you have in your kitchen, for example, broccoli, swede and cauliflower.

NOTE

You may need the addition of 1 tablespoon of water or white wine after sautéing. Continue cooking on a low heat until all the liquid has evaporated.

You can also add at this stage 1 tablespoon balsamic vinegar or the juice of half a lemon.

Cauliflower Rice
Serves 2 - 3

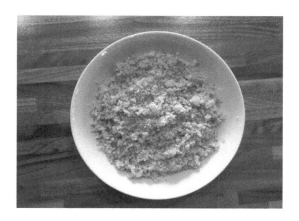

INGREDIENTS
1 large cauliflower cut up into small florets, including stalk as well
1 tablespoon of refined olive oil or coconut oil

METHOD
Pre heat oven to 180 C, Fan 160 C, 350 F, Gas 4.
Prepare your cauliflower.
Place cauliflower into a food processor (does not seem to work as well with a blender) and pulse cauliflower until it resembles 'rice' or 'couscous'.
At this stage you can use it straight away or spread it on a non-stick baking tray, place it into the oven for approximately 5 - 8 minutes.
DO NOT let it brown, keep stirring the cauliflower to mix it up. This slightly dries the cauliflower creating a drier type of rice.

TO COOK CAULIFLOWER RICE

Heat up oil of your choice in a wok or sauté pan.

Add in your cauliflower rice, fast fry for approximately 5 - 8 minutes, stirring continuously, then serve with a basic curry (this recipes can be found in the 'Dinners' section of this book).

VARIATIONS / ALTERNATES:

1. Fry a thinly sliced onion plus a few thinly sliced mushrooms in the heated oil, then add in 1 teaspoon of cumin seeds or 1 teaspoon of fennel seeds before adding in your cauliflower rice.
   For extra richness you can always add a knob of butter at the end.

2. Fry 1 clove of peeled and crushed garlic and 1 inch piece of fresh ginger, peeled and crushed in the heated oil, then you could add in cooked prawns or any leftover cooked meats etc.

Experiment with your compliant ingredients and create your own Special Fried Rice.

For Egg Fried Rice, we chop up a 2 egg cooked omelette. We add it after we have cooked the cauliflower rice at the end, to heat the egg through, remembering to stir thoroughly. It is really tasty and a great accompaniment to meat dishes.

NOTE

We have found out recently you can now buy prepared cauliflower rice from supermarkets, e.g. Aldi (in the vegetable section). It freezes really well and cooks from frozen!

Brilliant, always handy in case of last minute dinner guests.

Cauliflower Mash

Serves 4
Freezes well

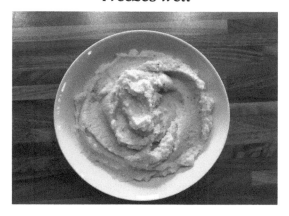

INGREDIENTS

2 medium/large cauliflowers cut into florets including stalks
50 grams butter cut into ½ inch cubes
Salt and pepper to taste
Good grating of fresh nutmeg. Pre-grated dried nutmeg can be used, but it is not as tasty.

METHOD

Prepare your ingredients.
Cook your cauliflowers in a large pan of boiling water until soft. (Can be steamed instead but it takes longer.)
Drain thoroughly when cooked, leave it for 1 - 2 minutes, until it dries out and no water is dripping off it.
Place cooked cauliflower in a food processor, (See note at end of recipe if you do not have a food processor) add butter and process it until it is very smooth.
Add salt, pepper, grate in nutmeg, mixing well.

This can be made ahead of when you need it. It is more manageable when cold i.e. it's a lot easier to spread.

VARIATION
For a spicy flavour:
Add a teaspoon of ground cumin at the same time you add the nutmeg
<u>Or</u>
Use 1 teaspoon Madras Curry Powder, instead of the nutmeg.

NOTE
If you do not have a food processor use either a stick blender or a potato hand masher. It will take a little longer.

Homemade Pesto Sauce

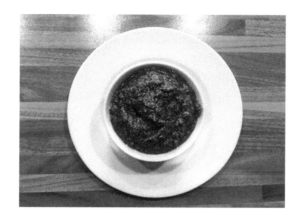

INGREDIENTS
2 generous handfuls of basil leaves including stalks
55 grams Parmesan cheese, finely grated
55 grams pine nuts
2 cloves of garlic, peeled
Juice of 1 lemon
150 ml Extra Virgin Olive oil
Salt and pepper to taste

METHOD
Wash and pat dry basil leaves, stalks, to remove the excess water.
Place basil, pine nuts, cheese, garlic, lemon juice, salt and pepper into a food processor or high powdered blender, and process ingredients until smooth.
We then add ¾ of the oil to the mixture, in case the mixture goes too runny!
Continue adding the oil a bit at a time, till you are happy with the consistency of the pesto sauce. Always taste it at this stage as it may need a little bit more salt.
To store, place your pesto sauce into an airtight container/jar in the fridge, it lasts 7 - 10 days.

NOTE

We use it as a marinade on vegetables. You can thin it down with more oil or vinegar as a pesto salad dressing.
Or as a topping on any of the following:
chicken
salmon/fish
pork tenderloin/chops,
beef burgers etc.

A dessertspoon of pesto sauce can be stirred/mixed in just before serving to any sautéed vegetables or your Cabbage Tagliatelle.

Basic Spice Mix

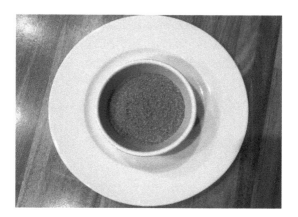

This can be used for all meat, fish and vegetable curries. At the end of this recipe there are slight additions and amendments for different curries and tastes.

INGREDIENTS

1 dessertspoon coriander powder
¾ dessertspoon cumin powder
½ teaspoon turmeric powder
¼ - ½ teaspoon garam masala powder
½ teaspoon chilli powder to your taste (we use hot chilli powder as we find it has a better taste).

METHOD

Place all the above ingredients into a mixing bowl, mixing thoroughly.
You can make this in double, treble or even greater quantities BUT always use the same ratios.
To store spice mix, keep in an airtight container, in the dark where it is cool.
Do not make too much as it can go off after a couple of months, losing its spicy flavour.

ADDITIONS AND AMENDMENTS

For nearly all curries we start by heating up the oil in whatever pan you are using and add 1 - 2 teaspoons of black mustard seeds, fry them until they start to 'pop'. Add onions, ginger and garlic as in our basic curry recipe, which can be found in the 'Dinners' section of this book.

Chicken Curries

Normally we just use the basic spice mix recipe, sometimes we add, as we start frying, 4- 5 crushed cardamom pods.

Lamb Curries

As you start frying, add 1 teaspoon of fenugreek powder, 1 teaspoon black mustard seeds, about 2 inches cinnamon bark, 4 - 5 whole cloves to the basic spice mix recipe.

Fish and Vegetables Curries

As you start frying, add 1 teaspoon black mustard seeds, 1 dessertspoon fennel seeds to the basic spice mix recipe.

Beef Curries

Add a couple of star anise when you fry your onions.

BOUGHT SPICE MIXTURES

CHECK the ingredients make sure they do not contain any rice, maize or corn flour. We find East End spices are really good.

NOTE

Play around with the spices in different ratios to find a mix that suits your taste, REMEMBER it is not all about heat! Some of the heat comes from the fresh ginger you use in curries. Spice and heat are not the same.
Spice is more important than heat.

We sometimes use curry leaves in our curries. You can buy them from Asian supermarkets.

To store them put in a zip lock freezer bag, place into freezer straight away. Take them out when you need them.

Can be used straight from frozen. We use 12 - 15 leaves per curry.

They add a lovely flavour, dried ones are ok but don't have the same flavour.

Homemade Nut Butters

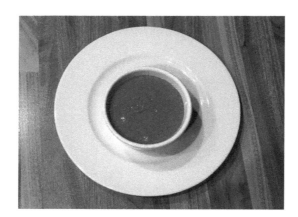

INGREDIENTS

1kg raw nuts, not salted
You can use almonds, macadamias, hazelnuts, Brazil, pistachio, or pecan nuts.
Walnuts can be used, however you need to remove their skins as they cause the
butter to have a slightly bitter taste.

NOTE

We find almonds, hazelnut and pecans are the best. Our favourite ratio is 700
grams almonds, plus 300 grams pecans. These seem to work best.

METHOD

Preheat oven to 200 C, Fan 180 C, 400 F, Gas 6
On an unlined baking tray, spread out almonds and pecans, place on middle shelf
of preheated oven.
Roast nuts for approximately 8 - 10 minutes, remember to mix them up halfway
through, and don't let them burn. (If this happens your butter will taste bitter.)
Remove from oven, leave them to cool on your baking tray, until almost cold
but not quite, very slightly warm to the touch. Then add your prepared nuts

in batches to a food processor or blender. On full power, blend prepared nuts until you have nut butter. This will take a good 10 -15 minutes usually (if using a blender you will need to press them down with the handle of a wooden spoon). At first it will look as though all you have got is nut dust but suddenly you will notice the oil beginning to form in the blender. Continue to blend/mix until quite smooth.

Almond makes a thicker butter, whereas the other nuts have a much looser consistency. This is because of the different oil contents in the nuts.

Place nut butter into an airtight container. We have found that it will keep for a month (if you can resist it). You do not need to keep it in the refrigerator. Serve and enjoy.

We have our nut butter on homemade flaxseed crackers or on a plate as a dip with vegetable crudités as a snack, or drizzle it over homemade sugar free vanilla ice cream. It is also fabulous mixed in with natural Greek, sheep's, or goat's yogurt.

There are lots of ways of eating nut butter - you will be surprised!

NOTE

Whilst we were experimenting to find different recipes of nut butters we altered the ratios of the nuts we use.

At first we halved them. We did a batch of 250 grams almonds plus 250 grams pecans. Then we tried 350 grams almonds plus 150 grams pecans. We continued until we found one that suited our tastes.

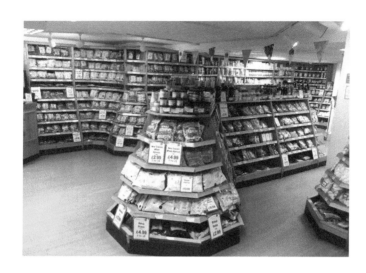

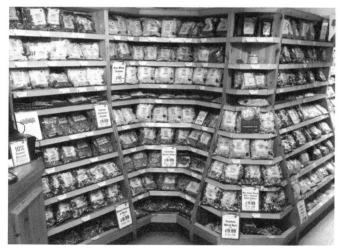

GrapeTree, packed with nuts and seeds.

DESSERTS

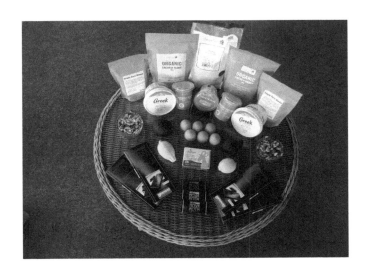

Cinnamon Bramley Apple Almond Pudding
Serves 8

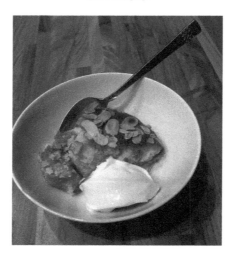

INGREDIENTS

2 large Bramley apples, peeled, cored, cut into wedges
1 teaspoon ground cinnamon
100 grams softened unsalted butter
3 large eggs, beaten
150 grams ground almonds
1 tablespoon almond extract
25 grams flaked almonds
50 grams stevia or sweetener of your choice

METHOD

Preheat oven to 190 C, Fan 170 C, 375 F, Gas 5
Prepare your ingredients.
Place butter and stevia into a bowl, whisk together until pale and fluffy.
Begin adding the eggs, little at a time, they could curdle if you add them too
quickly. (Note by having all ingredients at room temperature it helps to stop this

happening.) Add almond extract and fold in ground almonds, until all mixed in. Place apple wedges, teaspoon of sweetener and cinnamon into dish you are using. Spoon mixture over apples, levelling it out with the back of a spoon. Sprinkle flaked almonds over top of mixture.

Place dish on to a baking tray, put on middle shelf of preheated oven, for 30 - 35 minutes, or until pudding is golden on top and feels firm in the middle.

If your pudding seems to be browning too quickly, cover with a sheet of foil/parchment paper.

If your oven is cooking your pudding unevenly, turn once during cooking. Remove from oven and allow to cool slightly.

Divide into 8 portions; serve with double cream, crème fraîche or Greek yogurt.

VARIATIONS

You can swap 1 tablespoon almond extract, and replace with either 2 tablespoons vanilla extract or 10 grams ground ginger.

Also

If you would prefer a more fudge like filling, you can add 80 grams of homemade nut butter, see 'Side Dishes and Accompaniments' section of this book for the recipe.

Lemon Posset
Serves 4 - 6

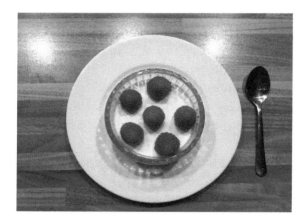

INGREDIENTS
Zest and juice of 2 lemons
500 ml Double Cream
10 grams Stevia or sweetener of your choice

METHOD
Add lemon zest, cream and stevia into a pan. On a medium heat, bring to a simmer. Heat until all the stevia has dissolved, stirring occasionally.
Remove pan from heat, immediately add in lemon juice and stir.
Allow mixture to cool, then using a sieve, pour mixture through sieve into a large jug. Straight away pour the mixture into 4 - 6 ramekins (depends on size of your ramekins, I use the little white ones).
Allow to cool at room temperature. Then cover each ramekin with a piece of cling film, place in fridge to set and leave them overnight.

SERVING
Bring out of fridge, uncover them and allow them to reach room temperature.
You can then serve them on their own, with fresh berries or even warm berries.
You can always swap lemons for limes, same amounts, same method used.

No Bake Lime Cheesecake
Serves 8

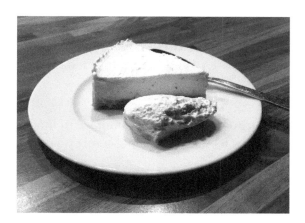

INGREDIENTS

Base
200 grams ground almonds
75 grams unsalted butter, softened
1 tablespoon melted coconut oil
5 grams stevia or sweetener of your choice

Filling
2 x 250 grams mascarpone cheese
5 grams stevia or sweetener of your choice
Zest and juice of full lime (use 2 limes if you like it tart)

METHOD

For the Base
Using a 7-inch spring base cake tin, line the bottom and sides of cake tin with cling film (this helps it to come out cleanly)
Combine the melted coconut oil and softened butter together with ground

almonds and stevia, and mix thoroughly. It should form a moist but fairly dry base - if mixture is too wet add a dessertspoon spoon of coconut flour a bit at a time, until you get the right consistency. Place mixture into base of prepared cake tin, press down with back of spoon until it is nice and level. Place cake tin into fridge until it sets.

For the Filling
Meanwhile place mascarpone cheese, zest and juice of lime or limes (depending on how tart you would like it) plus stevia into a mixing bowl and mix thoroughly.
Once base of your cheesecake is cool and set, spoon on filling, level with back of a spoon, leave overnight in fridge to set.

Serving
Remove from fridge and cake tin.
Leave it on kitchen side, until it reaches room temperature, then serve either alone, or with berries of your choice i.e. raspberries, strawberries, etc. You can also add whipped double cream, crème fraiche, or Greek yogurt.

VARIATIONS
For lemon cheesecake remove lime/limes from recipe and replace with lemon/lemons (depending how tart you like it).

NOTE
For a special occasion dessert, what I do is thinly slice strawberries and press them on the sides of the cheesecake, I also use 2 - 3 large strawberries with green top stalk left on, partially slice from base of each strawberry ¾ the way up towards the top, then fan each strawberry out to use them as centre decorations.

If any cheesecake is left place into an airtight box and keep in fridge.

Vanilla and Almond Sponge Cake
Serves 6 - 8

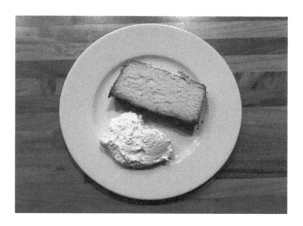

INGREDIENTS

175 grams unsalted softened butter
75 grams coconut flour
75 grams ground almonds
3 large eggs, beaten
75 grams stevia or sweetener of your choice
½ teaspoon baking powder
1 tablespoon vanilla extract

METHOD

Preheat oven to 180 C, Fan 160 C, 350 F, Gas 4
In a large bowl, place softened butter, sweetener of your choice and whisk until light and fluffy.
Whisk in beaten eggs to mixture, now add in the coconut and almond flours, baking powder, vanilla extract, keep whisking until all ingredients are combined. If mixture feels too thick, add up to 1 tablespoon of milk or almond milk. Spoon mixture into lined 2lb loaf tin, place on middle shelf in preheated oven.

Bake for 35 - 45 minutes or until golden brown and the middle feels firm, alternately you can insert a skewer into centre of cake, if it comes out clean, then it is cooked.
Place on cooling rack until cool, then remove from tin.
You can store it in an airtight container until you are ready to use.

Servings
It is delicious on its own, but even better with whipped double cream, crème fraiche or Greek yogurt. You can also add fresh berries.

VARIATIONS
You can replace Vanilla Extract with any of the following;
½ teaspoon coffee essence or
an espresso of strong black coffee or
juice and zest of 2 limes or
Juice and zest of 2 lemons or
100 grams 100% cocoa powder.

Death by Chocolate Cake
Serves 8 - 10

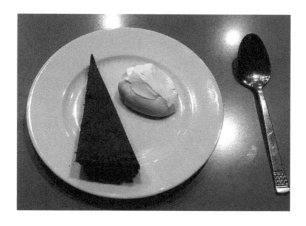

INGREDIENTS

350 grams dark chocolate (I use a mixture of 74% and 85% cocoa solids) broken into pieces
250 grams unsalted butter, cut into pieces
3 large eggs
50 grams stevia sweetener or a sweetener of your choice
75 grams coconut flour
1 teaspoon baking powder
Water or milk if mixture feels too thick

METHOD

Preheat the oven to 160 C, Fan 140 C, 325 F, Gas 3
Butter and line a 9-inch round cake tin. Melt the chocolate, butter together, (I usually do it in a microwave bowl, 30 seconds at a time until it has melted, keep checking it though), mix it well and leave to cool.
In a separate bowl, whisk the eggs, until pale, then whisk in the sweetener gradually until mixture is thick, glossy, well combined.

Gently fold in the cooled melted chocolate mixture, sift in the flour and baking powder, gently stirring until smooth.

Pour into prepared cake tin and bake for 30 - 40 minutes, or until firm to the touch. You can test this by inserting a skewer into the middle of it, if it comes out clean it's ready, if not, leave in oven for a few more minutes then check again. The mixture will be soft in the middle but as it cools it does firm up. Leave cake in tin, place on cooling rack for at least I hour. Serve the cake warm, or cold with whipped double cream. Delicious.

TREATS

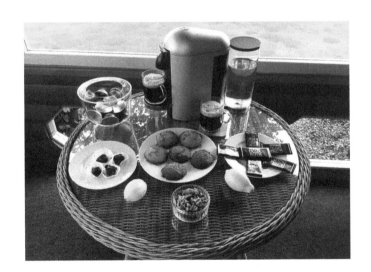

Sugar Free Raspberry, Almond, Coconut Ice Cream
Serves 8

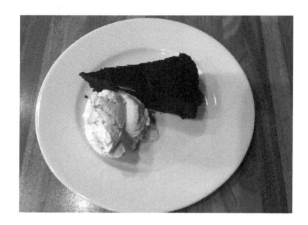

INGREDIENTS

500 ml coconut cream

250 ml unsweetened almond milk, freeze in ice cube tray before use.

2 teaspoons almond extract or to your taste

30 grams stevia or sweetener of your choice.

1 full punnet fresh raspberries, cut in pieces, open freeze on a plate, before use.

METHOD

You will need a blender.

Put ingredients into your blender in the same order as above. Make sure lid is on properly.

Blend on full power until mixture is smooth, if it rises up in the blender, press it back down with the handle of a wooden spoon.

Ice cream in blender should look like 4 pillows, one in each corner.

Do not over blend, otherwise you will end up with an extra thick smoothie!

Serve and enjoy.

Place remaining ice cream into an airtight container with lid and place in freezer.

Drop Scones
Makes 10

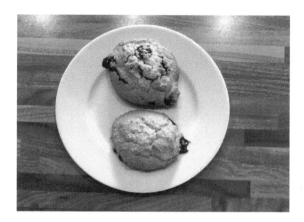

INGREDIENTS
300 grams almond flour or ground almonds
¼ teaspoon salt
½ teaspoon baking powder
2 large eggs, beaten
40 grams stevia or sweetener of your choice
115 grams unsalted butter, softened
90 grams fresh or frozen berries of your choice

METHOD
Preheat oven to 220 C, Fan 200 C, 425 F, Gas 7
Grease baking tray with butter or line with greaseproof paper. In a mixing bowl, mix together all the dry ingredients.
In a separate bowl, whisk eggs until light and fluffy.
Combine all dry and wet ingredients. Fold in berries of your choice.
I use an ice cream scoop to drop the dough mixture onto prepared baking tray (remember not too close as they may spread a little).

Bake in preheated oven, on middle shelf for 15 - 20 minutes or until scones have risen and are slightly brown.
Remove from oven, allow to cool and firm up for a few minutes, and then place on cooling rack. We like them warm with butter on them!
Serve and enjoy.

Chocolate Almond Butter Truffles
Makes 26

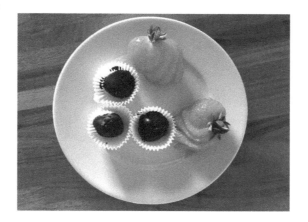

INGREDIENTS

200 grams Almond nut butter
(can be found under 'Side dishes and Accompaniments' section of this book)
50 - 75 grams almond flour (depends on consistency of nut butter you are using)
2 tablespoons stevia or sweetener of your choice
70 grams sugar free chocolate, (90% maximum cocoa solids)

METHOD

Place almond butter, sweetener, 50 grams almond flour into a bowl and blend until all combined.
If mixture is still quite runny, add in more almond flour, a teaspoon or tablespoon at a time, until mixture becomes dough like in consistency that can be rolled into balls.
Roll balls in to approximately 10 -12 grams size balls. (Makes 26 balls)
Break chocolate into small pieces, place into a microwave bowl, and then carefully microwave chocolate 30 seconds at a time until it has melted.

Using a spoon coat each ball in chocolate, place chocolate coated truffles on a prepared plate that has been covered with parchment paper.
Leave to set in fridge 20 minutes. Serve alone or with fruit and enjoy.

NOTE
These can be frozen for up to a month.
Remove from freezer 20 minutes before needed and leave to defrost at room temperature.

Extra 85% Dark Chocolate

Serves 1

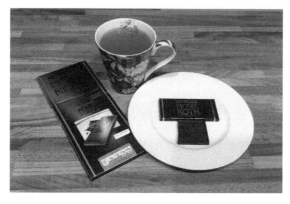

This is my naughty but nice treat!

INGREDIENTS

1½ small bars of 85% dark chocolate (74% dark chocolate is the minimum you should have)

NOTE

We buy our dark chocolate from Aldi as this particular bar comes with 5 individual wrapped bars that weigh 25 grams.
It is my treat and I don't have to share it!

METHOD

I always have chocolate in my drawer.
When a need a treat I either have 1 bar which to be truthful is plenty, but sometimes I just need more!
Sounds familiar?
If so, I make a cup of black earl grey tea, place my chocolate on a plate and sit where I can relax, without being disturbed, to thoroughly enjoy it!
Guess what?
It always works.

Chapter 15:
Daily diary example

Overleaf is a template of our daily food diary. Please feel free to photocopy this to complete yourselves, or alternatively, make and complete your own.

Following the template overleaf, there is an excerpt from our diary. It has been absolutely essential for us to be able to refer back too over the past year and a half.

It's reminded us to keep on track and it's also been great for looking back to eliminate any foods that have had a negative or bad reaction on our progress. We're sure you will all find yours helpful as well. Incidentally, we have kept ours even whilst on holiday. 'A bit over the top' I hear you say, but no, it really isn't. It's been both essential and a godsend.

Make sure you include the weights of your protein, i.e. meat, fish and cheese. Endeavour to keep within your protein limits. Remember, it's only 25 grams of cheese a day and 100 grams of meat or fish at any one serving. Depending how big your hands are, a handful of mixed nuts is between 30 - 50 grams, so keep an eye on how much you grab for your snacks.

On the diary sheet I have included a section called '**Additional information, notes and observations from that day.**' This section can be used to record your weight if you've been weighed that day, as well as any physical or mental observations, i.e. feeling down or upbeat, tired or full of energy, bloated etc. It's your diary, so put exactly how you're doing and feeling!

Also add any positive observations/ compliments you have received from other people that day.

They can be a real boost for you!

Daily Diary example

Day and Date	
Breakfast	
Lunch	
Snack	
Dinner (including dessert)	
Treats*	

* *(We would include our 25 grams of dark chocolate here.)*

Additional information, notes and observations from that day.

Example of an entry in our diary

Day and Date	Saturday 14th April
Breakfast	20 grams mixed nuts. 50 grams sheep's yogurt.
Lunch	Half an avocado. 20 grams mixed nuts. Stick of celery.
Snack	Small piece of homemade carrot cake.
Dinner (including dessert)	150 grams pan-fried salmon. (we had 150 grams of salmon as we did not have 100 grams of protein at lunch, otherwise it would be only 100 grams of salmon) Sautéed cabbage, kale and onion. 2 tablespoons olive oil.
Treats	25 grams 85% dark chocolate.

Additional information, notes and observations from that day.

After our first 3 weeks into our new lifestyle , we have both lost 1 stone each. Unbelievable - we both feel fantastic.

Very recently we had been looking through our diary to check on a few things that were not actually agreeing with our bodies.

This resulted in us having a conversation about wood burners!

It may sound strange, but, your gut can be quite closely compared to a wood burner.

If you feed the burner with good wood, such as Ash or Oak, it burns for a long time, cleanly. It has little smoke or toxic fumes and in the morning when you go to clean out the fire, there's very little ash or waste. However, if you burn a lot of unseasoned, damp or soft wood, it burns badly and very inefficiently, producing far less heat (energy) and tends to smoke a lot, blacken your fire glass and soot up your chimney. In the morning there's loads of ash and clinker in the bottom of the fire.

It's the same with your food.

If you eat and supply your gut with the best food you can, it provides sustained energy, without the sugar and insulin peaks that many other foods do and there's very little waste at the end of it all!

Also the process of digestion doesn't create lots of unwanted toxins that leech into your body, which in turn, can cause numerous everyday medical problems. I don't intend to go into these medical issues as I'm obviously not a doctor and have no scientific proof.

I will say however, from our own experience, you will notice some big differences in your body and how you will start feeling. The purpose of the conversation being to reinforce how important your daily diary is, in order to check back on what you're eating on a daily basis.

Chapter 16:
Fun and games with sweeteners

As I write this chapter, we find ourselves coming to the end of an experiment with sweeteners. We are currently in a friend's house in a sleepy village in southern Spain. We've travelled here in order to have some peace and quiet, away from all the usual distractions around us at home, in order to put the finishing touches to this book.

We've been away for six weeks now and during this time we have not eaten any baking, i.e. puddings, cakes or anything containing sugar or sweeteners. That is, apart from, a slight mistake with some bottled, skinned and de-seeded red peppers we thought were in olive oil. We added them to our salads, however, after several days we both began to feel really 'off'.

We put this 'off' feeling down to all sorts of causes. The local water. The hot weather. The local swimming pool. It was none of these though.

We checked our food diary and realised our 'off' feeling was down to the introduction of the red bottled peppers. It was all it could be. We checked the ingredients and guess what? They contain added sugars! We subsequently threw them away and just went back to our normal eating, again minus any baked goods and stevia. During the course of the next eight hours we immediately started feeling fine again.

A further study of our diary told us that prior to going to Spain, Julie had been experimenting with her baking and using a fair amount of stevia. We had begun to experience hunger during that time again. Something we hadn't done for the previous twelve months!

Whilst in Spain this had disappeared again completely. We weren't hungry between meals anymore.

Our Conclusion

We really believe that stevia as well as other so called natural sweeteners mess with your mind and body, triggering off those responses that make you always feel hungry. Even though it's supposed to be zero calories and zero carbs, the sweetness is what triggers off the responses in your body!

This is something we are definitely going to keep a very close watch on in the future. Obviously we don't have any real scientific proof of this but there is plenty on the Internet that suggests that does occur. Food labels are the other things we are going to watch closely. Always have a good look at them if you're unsure what is in the jars or can!

Chapter 17:
Our final parting words. For now!

Our Final Parting Words

IF YOU HAVE GOT THIS FAR THEN YOU HAVE READ ALL ABOUT OUR INCREDIBLE
JOURNEY

We hope you have tried some of our recipes as well as experimented with a few of your own
favourite family versions.

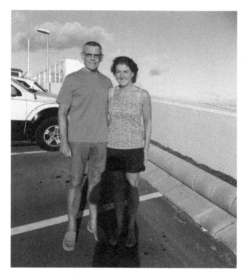

By now you will feel like us: "A Million Dollars"
Healthier,
Loads more energy,
Less stressed,
Sleeping better,
Toned up,
Definitely younger looking!

Wouldn't it be great if we could bottle these feelings and SPRINKLE them onto our loved ones, friends and
doubting Thomases, so they all could benefit like we have!

KEEP UP THE GOOD WORK and ENJOY YOUR LIFE, IT IS REALLY WORTH IT!!

<u>REMEMBER IT'S NOT WHAT YOU EAT BUT WHAT YOU DON'T EAT THAT MATTERS!</u>

Acknowledgments and Thanks

We would like to give a big thank you to both Lakeland and Booths supermarket for their help and allowing us to take photographs of their premises and produce.

We would also like to thank Grape Tree for allowing us to take photographs of their store in Skipton. They are always our first choice for our nuts, seeds, herbs, alternative flours and sweeteners. They also have an excellent on line service.

Thank you to all our friends and family who have offered their support and advice throughout the writing of this book. A bigger thank you goes to all the doubting Thomas's who told us we were wasting our time. They actually helped to spur us on to completing the book.

Corny, but necessary, we need to thank each other for the constant support we've given each other. Big hugs all round!

Thanks to Annie and Rafe for making sure it all made sense.

Thanks to Catherine Cousins and the team at 2QT Publishing, who made our dream into what you are reading.

Finally we need to mention Apple, and in particular their store in Leeds, for their brilliant help and advice in putting everything together. Their studio sessions have been invaluable. They have been superb and we cannot recommend them highly enough. In particular, Ross, Ian, Rachel and Dan.

Anyone needing advice or embarking on a project themselves will benefit massively from the sessions.

About the Authors

Julie and Martin Carrick are down to earth Yorkshire people. They are both originally from Sheffield and now reside in the Yorkshire Dales near Settle. They have two grown up boys, who are both married.

They are both former Police Officers and are now retired.

Neither of them are writers, authors or experts on nutrition. They are just ordinary folk who have a passion for life and an even greater passion for food and cooking.

They are both keen motorcyclists and can be often found on the roads around the Dales and the Lake District, as well as venturing across the water into other parts of Europe, usually in search of some sun! Talking of sun, they travel a fair bit and enjoy trying the local food wherever they find themselves.

This book shares their journey on a completely different eating experience than they were accustomed to previously, in an effort to lose weight and become healthier.

They've certainly achieved great success and believe that other people will be very interested in achieving and sharing that same success!

Now is the time for you to join them on their journey!

Contact Us

By email: julieandmartinlosingit@gmail.com

By Facebook - search 'Losing it with Julie and Martin'

Index for Recipes

Side Dishes and Accompaniments

Desserts

Treats